Charles Bonnet Syndrome and Other Visual Hallucinations

This book examines Charles Bonnet Syndrome and other visual hallucinations beyond the basic neuroscience concepts by providing the reader with a prevailing clinically applicable overview. It is a practical guide for those clinicians assessing patients who present with visual hallucinations and require additional evaluation to make a diagnosis and helps the clinician to formulate a clear management approach. In addition, there is a useful narrative section with multiple case analyses that assists clinicians, current patients, and their caregivers to understand how others have personally dealt with these problems and which treatment modality has worked best for them.

Key Features:

- Discusses medical, surgical, optical and psychological treatment plans.
- Appeals to practising neuro-ophthalmologists, ophthalmologists, optometrists, low-vision specialists, neurologists, psychologists, psychiatrists, occupational/physical therapists and rehabilitation counsellors.
- Uses multiple clinical cases and scenarios as illustrative examples.
- Uses current technology to illustrate visual hallucinations as seen by patients.
- Can be used as a teaching tool for the patient and their caregiver.

Charles Bonnet Syndrome and Other Visual Hallucinations

Clinical Diagnosis and Management

Edited by
Leonid Skorin, Jr.
Gary M. Cusick

CRC Press
Taylor & Francis Group
Boca Raton London New York

CRC Press is an imprint of the
Taylor & Francis Group, an **informa** business

Designed cover image: Stefano Cena

First edition published 2026
by CRC Press
2385 NW Executive Center Drive, Suite 320, Boca Raton FL 33431

and by CRC Press
4 Park Square, Milton Park, Abingdon, Oxon, OX14 4RN

CRC Press is an imprint of Taylor & Francis Group, LLC

ISBN: 978-1-041-05996-7 (hbk)
ISBN: 978-1-041-05986-8 (pbk)
ISBN: 978-1-003-63336-5 (ebk)

DOI: 10.1201/9781003633365

Typeset in Sabon
by SPi Technologies India Pvt Ltd (Straive)

Access the Resource Center: https://resourcecentre.routledge.com/books/9781041059868

This book is dedicated to four individuals who were instrumental in my training and career:

- Bruce E. Onofrey, RPh, OD, who was my optometry college classmate and whose intellect I tried to emulate. Later becoming my co-author, co-editor, co-lecturer and, most importantly, my friend.
- Richard F. Multack, DO, OD, MBA, who was my ocular disease professor in optometry college and directed me to medicine. Later becoming a mentor during my osteopathic medical college training and beyond.
- Jeffrey N. Holtzman, DO, who was my ophthalmology residency program director and taught me how to be a skilled ophthalmic surgeon, just like he was, while always treating me like a son.
- James A. Goodwin, MD, who was my neuro-ophthalmology fellowship director and a brilliant diagnostician and taught me how to disentangle the mysteries of neuro-ophthalmic disease.

—L.S.

To my local support: Debra, Helen, Zora, and Patricia
Out of town support: Eva and Shaimond
And the Saturday Support Group

—G.M.C.

Contents

Preface

> "It is much simpler to buy books than to read them, and easier to read them than to absorb their contents."[1]
>
> **–Sir William Osler**

Charles Bonnet Syndrome (CBS) was first described by its eponymist, the Swiss philosopher, biologist and naturalist Charles Bonnet, in his book *Essai Analytique sur les Facultés de L'âme* in 1760.[2] However, the term itself does not appear in print until 1936.[3] In that year, a Geneva neurologist, Georges de Morsier, published a brief article on visual hallucinations and coined the term we use today.

With this long history, how is it that in modern medical publications one still finds terms such as misdiagnosed, misinterpreted, underestimated, underreported, unrecognized, underdiagnosed, and overlooked still being applied to CBS? Before 1990 CBS was even considered a rare occurrence.[4] There appear to be many potential explanations that may confound CBS terminology and definition. These include the addition of labels such as pseudohallucination, the fact that no universal standardized criteria exist, that exclusion criteria are not uniform across scientific studies, and that the patients themselves are afraid to confess to "seeing things." Reaching even further back, de Morsier himself fumbled with the terminology and redefined CBS a couple of times, from his original paper in 1936 to his latter publication on the topic in 1967.[5]

Besides the above-stated issues, another problem is that although there is now more information about CBS, this information, being oriented to the neuroscientist, is less clinical and more theoretical. This is why the idea of compiling a comprehensive source that covers all the current thinking, including the misconceptions about CBS, and then incorporating and applying clinical relevance to it came about. *Charles Bonnet Syndrome and Other Visual Hallucinations: Clinical Diagnosis and Management* has been designed for those clinicians who see these patients. It provides the clinicians with the tools necessary to accurately diagnose, counsel, treat, and refer these patients when indicated, for other helpful resources. As a bonus, not only does almost every chapter conclude with a representative patient case, but the last chapter of this book is composed of numerous illustrative patient case reports by a myriad of various clinicians detailing their CBS patient experiences and how they diagnosed, counseled and addressed the patients' visual hallucinations.

If you are reading this Preface, you have already progressed through the first two steps of Dr. Osler's epigram. Now, as you continue to read the following chapters of this book, we sincerely hope that when you finish, you will have also achieved his final step by absorbing their contents.

Leonid Skorin, Jr.
Gary M. Cusick

REFERENCES

1. Osler W, The Medical Library in Post-Graduate Work: An address delivered at the Inaugural Meeting of the Medical Library Association. *Proceedings of the Medical Library Association*, Vol. I, Part II. London: British Medical Association; 1909:14. https://archive.org/details/b22426711/page/14/mode/2up?ref=ol&view=theater. Accessed July 29, 2025.
2. Bonnet C, *Essai Analytique sur les Facultés de L'âme*. Copenhagen: Freres Cl. & Ant. Philbert; 1760:315–7.
3. de Morsier G, Les automatismes visuels. Hallucinations retrochiasmatiques. *Schweiz Med Wochenschr.* 1936;66: 700–8.
4. Sacks O, *Hallucinations*. New York: Alfred A. Knopf; 2012: 3–33.
5. de Morsier G, Le Syndrome de Charles Bonnet: Hallucinations visuelles des vieillards sans déficience mentale. *Ann Méd Psychol.* 1967;125: 677–702.

Acknowledgements

A special acknowledgement and thank you to all the contributors to the various chapters in this book and to the publisher for all their help in its publication.

Finally, we would specifically like to thank Shivangi Pramanik for believing in our book and Kanchi Shridhar for assistance with the editorial process.

Editor Biographies

Dr. Leonid Skorin, Jr. is meritoriously retired from the Mayo Clinic Health System in Albert Lea and Austin, MN where he was a Consultant in the Department of Surgery, Community Division of Ophthalmology. He was also an Assistant Professor of Ophthalmology at the Mayo Clinic College of Medicine and Science in Rochester, MN.

His degrees include a Doctor of Optometry from the Illinois College of Optometry and a Doctor of Osteopathic Medicine and Surgery from the Chicago College of Osteopathic Medicine. He did his medical/surgical internship in Tulsa, OK and his ophthalmology residency at Michigan State University/Metropolitan Hospital. He did a neuro-ophthalmology fellowship at the University of Illinois Eye & Ear Infirmary.

Dr. Skorin is a past president of the Minnesota Osteopathic Medical Society. He is a Costin Institute Scholar in osteopathic medical education and received the Presidential Achievement Certificate from the American Osteopathic College of Ophthalmology for his medical and surgical mission work in Ukraine. He has presented over 700 invited and named lectures throughout the United States, Canada, Australia, New Zealand, Spain, England, Germany and Ukraine. These included presentations at various optometry and osteopathic medical colleges. He has served as the Director and Chair of Continuing Medical Education at the Mayo Clinic Health System-Albert Lea, Minnesota Osteopathic Medical Society and the American Osteopathic College of Ophthalmology. He has several hundred scientific publications, including various textbook chapters. He is the Co-Editor and Co-Author of seven ophthalmic textbooks. He has served as a reviewer, columnist, member of the Board of Consultants for various professional journals and as both the Editor-In-Chief and the International Editor-In-Chief for the *Clinical & Surgical Journal of Ophthalmology*. In 2006, he was awarded the Distinguished Clinician of the Year Award from the Mayo Clinic Health System—Albert Lea. In 2016, he was named Mayo Clinic School of Health Sciences NP/PA Emergency Medicine Fellowship Program—Educator of the Year. He has trained osteopathic ophthalmology residents at the Chicago College of Osteopathic Medicine and was a preceptor for osteopathic medical and optometry students. In 2017, the American Osteopathic College of Ophthalmology awarded him the Governor's Achievement Certificate.

Dr. Skorin completed the Mayo Clinic/University of Minnesota Carlson School of Management Leadership Development Program in 2010 and a Master of Science in Medical Education Leadership through the University of New England College of Osteopathic Medicine in 2011. He completed the American Osteopathic Association Health Policy Fellowship in 2012. Dr. Skorin is a Fellow of the American Academy of Optometry and the American Osteopathic College of Ophthalmology.

Currently, Dr. Skorin teaches ophthalmology track courses at several osteopathic medical colleges, continues to present lectures and hands-on wet-labs at medical and optometry conferences, and is the medical director and a board member of the Charles Bonnet Syndrome non-profit support group, Mary Carmel's Light.

Dr. Gary M. Cusick is a Clinical Psychologist in Louisville Kentucky. His degrees and adult work have focused on working with persons with disabilities. His degrees include Masters in Rehabilitation Counselling from the University of Kentucky, and Doctor of Philosophy in Rehabilitation Psychology from the University of Wisconsin-Madison. His clinical work has included nursing homes, rehabilitation hospitals, and telehealth psychology clients.

His first experience with Charles Bonnet Syndrome (CBS) came while he was working at the Charles W. McDowell Blind Rehabilitation Center in Louisville. Now retired, he works with persons with CBS individually and hosts a weekly support group.

Contributors

Jesse Britt
Post-Graduate Year 1, Transitional Year
Madigan Army Medical Center
Tacoma, Washington

and

Flight Surgeon, 1st Aviation Brigade
Fort Novosel, Alabama

Stefano Cena
Department of Research
Rocky Vista University College of Osteopathic Medicine
Ivins, Utah

and

Graduate Research Scholar
Ann & Robert H. Lurie Children's Hospital of Chicago
Chicago, Illinois

Meagan Chapman
Occupational Therapist
Low Vision Works of Florida
Sarasota, Florida

Zachary Dwyer
A.T. Still University Kirksville College of Osteopathic Medicine
Kirksville, Missouri

Denise Goodwin
Professor of Optometry
Pacific University College of Optometry
Forest Grove, Oregon

Anmol Gosai
Lincoln Memorial University – DeBusk College of Osteopathic Medicine
Harrogate, Tennessee

Gregory Gosdigian
Lincoln Memorial University – DeBusk College of Osteopathic Medicine
Knoxville, Tennessee

James Hall
Retina Consultants of Carolina, P.A.
Spartanburg, South Carolina

Jeffrey Holt
Holt Eye Clinic
Hot Springs, Arkansas

Jasmyne Jenkins
Edward Via College of Osteopathic Medicine – Carolinas
Spartanburg, South Carolina

Andrew Krein
Devon Eye Clinic
Devon, Alberta, Canada

Donald Morris
South Hills Eye Associates
Pittsburgh, Pennsylvania

John F. Renfro
Retina Consultants of Carolina, P.A.
Spartanburg, South Carolina

Charlie Saccarelli
President, Chadwick Optical, Inc.
Schwenksville, Pennsylvania

Karen Squier
Associate Professor of Optometry
Chief of Low Vision Services
Southern College of Optometry
Memphis, Tennessee

Emily Stiles
Edward Via College of Osteopathic Medicine – Carolinas
Spartanburg, South Carolina

Smaran Teru
Post-Graduate Year 1, Ophthalmology
Henry Ford Health System
Detroit, Michigan

Chapter 1

INTRODUCTION

Leonid Skorin, Jr. and Gary M. Cusick

"The imagination must be given not wings but weights."[1]

—**Henry Adams**

Hallucinations are fascinating. As a neuro-ophthalmologist, visual hallucinations and their accomplices, illusions, are the most fascinating of all the various sensory distortions people can experience. As luck would have it, surveys of the general population have found that visual hallucinations are the most frequently occurring of all the different types of hallucinations.[2] Please note that, although I may be an avid fan of these visual phenomena, I do not necessarily support or excuse how these visual phenomena can cause anxiety, trepidation and mental anguish in patients who experience them. Therefore, as the epigram implies, as clinicians we should help first corral and then subdue our patients' "imaginations." For without imagination, there could be no visual hallucinations.

I have had multiple patients who I have seen and treated for chronic migraines through the use of botulinum toxin injections and osteopathic manipulation. Many of these patients, and others whom I have seen for ocular surgery consultation in my general ophthalmology clinic, have had a history of migraines with aura (classic migraines). Migraine with aura occurs in 15% to 30% of migraineurs.[3–5] Of all the migraineurs who experience an aura, visual disturbances such as visual hallucinations occur in 90% of these patients.[3] These visual aura can be simple unformed hallucinations such as spots, wavy lines, shimmering, arcs of light, zigzag lines or geometric ones such as webs, lattice formation, spirals, pinwheels, etc.[3, 6–8] The more complex formed hallucinations are metamorphopsia, micropsia, macropsia, teleopsia, pelopsia, microsomatognosia, macrosomatognosia and mosaic vision.[3, 6–8]

Personally, I have never experienced any of those types of visual hallucinations since I am not a migraineur. But I have experienced another form of visual hallucination. It only occurred once, yet I have always remembered the event. I was a young child of around five years of age. I was ill and running a high fever. I remember quite vividly lying in bed with my mother sitting on the bed beside me and consoling me. There they were, seeming as real as they could be, human skeletons flying down upon me. In addition, the walls of the bedroom began toppling down, and I had the sense that I was about to be crushed and buried beneath them. I remember turning over onto my stomach and hiding my head beneath the bed pillows, but to no avail. I could still see the skeletons and the

DOI: 10.1201/9781003633365-1

collapsing walls. How it all resolved is a lost memory. At this point in my life, that has been my one and only visual hallucinatory experience. And yet, this one event has remained with me for many decades. I can only imagine how those who have these types of visual hallucinations repeatedly for many days, weeks, months or even years may feel.

It was not just my personal visual hallucinatory experience that encouraged and propelled me to bring some practical clinical clarity to this topic. More importantly, it was my patients' striking and often lucid recollections of their own ongoing encounters and struggles with their visual hallucinations that spurred me on. In addition, my years of studying and investigating these phenomena compelled me to assemble this information.

But why single out Charles Bonnet Syndrome (CBS)? Certainly, what I personally experienced was not CBS. After migraine-related visual auras, CBS is the second most commonly presenting visual hallucination in my practice. Studies show that in clinical settings CBS is still frequently underdiagnosed and even misdiagnosed.[9, 10] I teach osteopathic medical students, physician assistants, nurse practitioners and optometry interns. I am always surprised to find that some of these trainees may have never heard of, let alone ever interviewed, a CBS patient. Whenever one of these trainees encounters a CBS patient in my practice, I encourage them to take the extra time to interview this patient and then do further study of CBS. This has resulted in several of the trainees publishing either articles or case reports in the scientific literature.[11] I had an optometry intern who saw his first CBS patient in my practice on his first day of a scheduled three-month clinical rotation. He was not familiar with CBS so I assigned him to gather all the CBS patients who we would see over his three months with me and write up their cases. He saw a total of six patients with CBS over the period. He and I co-authored an article on visual hallucinations and reviewed all six CBS case presentations (Original article available as an online resource in Ancillary material section of Chapter 1).[12] I felt that this scientific article had such significant clarity that I used it as a teaching instrument for future students and as a patient education tool. Patients and their caregivers all seemed so thankful and relieved when I gave them a copy of this article. They were happy to have a solid diagnosis with an official medical name and the six case presentations reassured them that they were not alone. I hope this book can now be a similar clinical and patient educational tool.

The patients in our article ranged from 69 to 100 years of age. The various underlying ocular pathologies included non-exudative (dry) macular degeneration, geographic macular atrophy, exudative (wet) macular degeneration, end-stage pseudoexfoliative glaucoma, end-stage chronic glaucoma, non-ischemic hemiretinal vein occlusion, central retinal vein occlusion, central retinal artery occlusion, proliferative diabetic retinopathy and advanced cataracts. Some of the patients had multiple etiologies of those listed above, resulting in significant vision loss. As expected, the visual hallucinations these patients experienced varied considerably. The summarized highlights of our six cases from the article are available as an online resource in the Ancillary material section of Chapter 1.

In those cases where an individual cannot distinguish whether the visual hallucination is real or unreal hallucinatory imaginary, they are likely to be labeled as out of contact with reality and therefore pathological.[13] Such a label is not appropriate for patients who have CBS visual hallucinations. The imagery is certainly "coming" from the brain, but the initiating pathology (etiology) originates either in the eyes or along the visual pathway. This is why the term pseudohallucination has been applied to CBS by some researchers.[14, 15] A true visual hallucination is experienced as objective and located in external space.[13] The pseudohallucination has been defined as either a hallucinatory experience that lacks strong realistic qualities were the individual does not consider the images as being real, or as subjectively experienced images of great vividness and clarity.[14] The neurologist Oliver Sacks defines pseudohallucinations as being "...not projected into external space." Rather, "they are seen, so to speak, on the inside of one's eyelids."[16] He and other authors have labeled them as inner hallucinations and verify that they possess all the other hallmarks of visual hallucinations.[16, 17]

As one can see from these definitions, CBS visual phenomena actually have key elements of both pseudohallucinations and true hallucinations. These would include being located in the external space, either occupying the whole visualized space or superimposed upon a portion of the real scene behind or around the hallucinatory imagery and knowing the images are not real and, in many instances, having great vividness and clarity of the imaginary scene. Therefore, these semantics appear to just muddle things more. The definition of hallucination itself may occasionally be unstable; not to mention that the language of description is frankly not specific enough to distinguish between these two concepts.[17] Consequently, it is not surprising that the usefulness of the distinction between true hallucinations and pseudohallucinations has been questioned and even rejected by various authors.[17, 18]

The relationship between true hallucinations and pseudohallucinations remains obscure; since the term pseudohallucination as it pertains to CBS appears to be potentially unsalvageable, it should be abandoned.[17] The final definitive definition for CBS has not yet been written.[19] Even the neurologist Georges de Morsier, who coined the eponym CBS in 1936, returned to it in 1967 and essentially redefined and reconfirmed the reality of the existence of CBS.[20, 21]

One final point of interest regarding CBS is that Charles Bonnet himself, later in his life, experienced the very visual hallucinations that bear his name. There is a myriad of eponyms named after clinicians and scientists in medicine. It is indeed a rare and possibly singular case where the eponymist actually gets too "live" the disorder that conveys his name. Supposedly, Charles Bonnet had been deaf from the age of seven.[21, 22] In his mid-20s he caught an eye illness which made it painful for him to maintain a clear focus for any extended period of time.[19] Eventually, he also developed cataracts, which degraded his vision even further. This caused him to switch from doing microscope-related entomological research to studying plant life, then psychology, and, finally, metaphysics.[19, 23] Later in life, when he was nearly blind, Bonnet started seeing strange images—similar symptomatology that he had written about in his earlier career.[19, 22] This was confirmed by his biographer who stated that Charles Bonnet saw "a number of fantastic objects which he recognized as illusory".[24]

—Leonid Skorin, Jr.

"Yesterday, upon the stair
I met a man who wasn't there
He wasn't there again today
I wish, I wish he'd go away...[25]"

—Hughes Mearns

Mearns's poem expresses the paradoxical nature of Charles Bonnet Syndrome. A phantom person appears that has depth, color, movement, and a hint of intention. It is fleeting and intangible so the client reasons that the person seen is not real. Repetition of this experience for months, however, can erode confidence in one's lucidity. How can your mind assess your mind's functioning? Isn't this measuring with a potentially "bent ruler"?

As a clinical psychologist, I am concerned with the possibility of the client falling down the rabbit hole and losing the ability to cope in the real world. Anxiety and isolation in CBS can become exaggerated and impact quality of life and daily functioning.[26] Early reassurance from providers that CBS is not mental illness is crucial to maintain faith in one's mental health.[27]

At the blindness training center where I worked for nearly two decades, I would occasionally hear my blind coworkers talking about CBS. An elderly woman would see the ground covered with flowers everywhere she went. Other than a fall hazard, it didn't sound too serious.

One afternoon a 40ish client with rod and cone dystrophy told me she was seeing cobwebs and distorted faces leering at her. She was clearly distressed about this. This was my first real experience working with a person with CBS. I had no idea where to start or how to help her.

I did my due diligence and read everything I could find on CBS. The first step appeared to be to referral to a support group. I think of myself as a good Googler, but I couldn't find a support group anywhere in the United States.

A call to Judith Potts of Esme's Umbrella in London, UK provided a model for assisting people with CBS. At this point, I began gently asking everyone I worked with if they were seeing things others could not see. About one in three were forthcoming about their experience. These were all working age adults, not just the elderly that were discussed in the medical journals.

My clients reported the random appearance of flashes of light, colors, shapes, patterns, parts of animals and people, to complete person/images. Some experienced immersive CBS in which the person seems to have been transported to a different location.[28] Reactions to CBS ranged from mild amusement to disabling anxiety causing disruption in daily living.

My primary concern is the level of belief a person with CBS may have regarding the reality of a person/image. People/images cause the greatest disturbance perhaps due to the emotional response they evoke. There is also a greater possibility of wanting to interact with complex people/images than with simple images.

Over-involvement with a CBS person/image can lead to a strongly held belief that what they see is real. People with CBS may talk to it frequently assigning personality or forming a relationship with the image. The person with CBS may imagine that the person/image is soundlessly communicating. With daily repetition, the person with CBS may develop an emotional investment in the person/image. Ultimately, the person/image may be reinterpreted as if it were a real entity rather than a consequence of sight loss.

Some support group participants will assign names to recurring person/images. Value judgment about the person/images are made with some person/images being "good" and others "bad". I have heard support group participants will enlist the help of the good person/images to control or run off the bad. This may provide a structure to think about what they perceive, or the beginnings of a strongly held belief.

A strongly held belief is a conviction that a person is deeply committed to.[29] Like a conspiracy theory, a strongly held belief may be supported by one's reference group. This belief has not become a delusion in that it is somewhat open to interpretation and may vary over time. Very few people with CBS will transition to delusional belief.

Arranging life around the person/images and their intuited intentions has been reported however, suggesting the strongly held belief has progressed to delusional level. Arguments with alarmed caregivers may ensue, but despite hard feelings, safety must be the first concern. Compassion for uncontrolled image experiences is encouraged.

With the emergence of CBS, the person's startle sensitivity, intrusive thoughts and level of arousal all increase. Rumination and vigilance can increase threat related thinking.[30] Coping with CBS requires a different mode of thinking to reduce the number of episodes and disturbance. The images must be devalued in terms of importance to one's life. To do so, observation of one's thinking processes is required.

Many of those in the support group report that attention to family and visitors, daily living needs, and personally meaningful pursuits can disrupt the cycle of images and distress.[31] In contrast, activation of the brain's default network in states such as mind wandering is related to increased production of internally created images.[32, 33]

Support group participants have claimed to see and hear CBS images simultaneously. To date, all people with this experience also have hearing impairment. One participant reported that the auditory component disappeared when he was wearing his hearing aids.

Research on multimodal hallucinations is limited to people with schizophrenia; thus, generalizing this data to people with CBS is questionable at best.[33] People with CBS are continually trying to put meaning to the images. It can be difficult to separate what the person truly hears, and what they deduce the images are saying. Often the people/images are moving their mouths, and the person may "remember" what they said after the fact.

Several recent articles confuse the definition of CBS. Some articles will call an auditory hallucination "Auditory Charles Bonnet Syndrome" even when no vision loss is present.[34–36] This is not Charles Bonnet Syndrome.

CBS occupies a unique position between medical and behavioral phenomena. It is not a mental illness but, if unaddressed, it may induce depression and anxiety. With the significant loss of vision that precedes the onset of CBS, sense of self can suffer. The ability to work, travel independently, and engage in meaningful activities declines in tandem with vision loss. People with CBS may have to simultaneously learn blindness skills while they are coping with anxiety, depression, and images.

Behavioral health professional treatment such as cognitive behavior therapy for serious distress over CBS images may be required following the physician's best effort. The demand for expertise in working with this population however is commensurate with the small percentage of visually impaired in the U.S.A. (~2%).[37] The Foundation Fighting Blindness, however, seeks to remedy a lack mental health resources appropriate for people with sight loss.[38]

With the scarcity of behavioral health professionals trained to work with visually impaired CBS individuals, support groups can fill the need for first-line care. Communication with others with CBS can suggest coping strategies and make the experience less isolating. Collaboration with consumer groups, non-profits, and state services may speed development of support groups throughout the United States.

My Zoom support group is now over five years old and includes participants from British Columbia to Florida. I speak to people with CBS and their caregivers seeking information many times each week by phone. Collaborators have created a podcast (https://cbsyndromepodcast.com/) and a 501(c)(3) (https://marycarmelslight.com/) to expand awareness of CBS. This outreach has engendered new support groups in North America.

An additional five clinical case vignettes are available as an online resource in the Ancillary material section of Chapter 1.

—Gary M. Cusick

REFERENCES

1. Levenson JC, et al., *The Letters of Henry Adams*, Vol. 5. Cambridge, MA: Belknap Press of Harvard Univ. Press; 1982–1988: 606.
2. Tien AY, Distribution of hallucinations in the population. *Soc Psych Psychiatric Epidemiol.* 1991;26: 287–92.
3. Green MW, Patients with headaches and neurologic features. In: Tepper SJ, Sheftell FD, Rapoport AM, eds, *The Spectrum of Migraine*. New York: McMahon Pub. Group; 2002: 58–64.
4. Burde RM, et al., *Clinical Decisions in Neuro-Ophthalmology*, 3rd edn. St. Louis: Mosby; 2002: 114–35.
5. Robbins L, Skorin L, Migraine headache. In: Onofrey BE, Skorin L, Holdeman NR, eds, *Ocular Therapeutics Handbook: A Clinical Manual*, 4th edn. Philadelphia: Wolters Kluver; 2020: 606–9.
6. Rizzo M, et al., Central disorders of visual function. In: Miller NR, Newman NJ, eds, *Walsh & Hoyt's Clinical Neuro-Ophthalmology*, 6th edn. Philadelphia: Lippincott Williams & Wilkins; 2005: 575–645.
7. Onofrj M, et al., The clinical association of visual hallucinations. In: Collerton D, Mosimann UP, Perry E, eds, *The Neuroscience of Visual Hallucinations*. Oxford: Wiley Blackwell; 2015: 91–117.
8. Davidoff R, *Migraine: Manifestations, Pathogenesis, and Management.* Philadelphia: F.A. Davis Co; 1995: 44–76.
9. Teunisse RJ, et al., Visual hallucinations in psychologically normal people: Charles Bonnet Syndrome. *Lancet.* 1996;347: 794–7.
10. Norton-Willson I, et al., Visual perceptual disorders resembling the Charles Bonnet Syndrome. A study of 434 consecutive patients referred to a psychogeriatric unit. *Fam Pract.* 1987;4: 27–35.
11. Soofi T, et al., Why is this patient having visual hallucinations? *J Am Acad Physic Assist.* 2018;31(1): 55–6.
12. Skorin L, et al., Charles Bonnet Syndrome: visual perception as deception. *Clin Surg Ophthalmol.* 2004;22(9): 242–52.
13. Aleman A, et al., *Hallucinations: The Science of Idiosyncratic Perception.* Washington, DC: American Psychological Association; 2009: 25–46.
14. Taylor FK, On pseudo-hallucinations. *Psychol Med.* 1981;11: 265–71.
15. Sims A, et al., Descriptive phenomenology. In: Gelder MG, Lopez-Ibor JJ, Andreasen NC, eds, *New Oxford Textbook of Psychiatry*. Oxford: Oxford Medical Pub; 2000: 55–70.
16. Sacks O, *Hallucinations*. New York: Alfred A. Knopf; 2012: x–xi; 12–15; 262–5.
17. Berrios GE, *The History of Mental Symptoms: Descriptive Psychopathology Since the Nineteenth Century*. Cambridge, UK: Cambridge University Press; 1996: 35–70.
18. Bentall RP, *Madness Explained: Psychosis and Human Nature*. London: Penguin Books; 2003: 347–77.

19. Draaisma D, *Disturbances of the Mind.* New York: Cambridge Univ. Press; 2009: 11–39.
20. de Morsier G, Les automatismes visuels. Hallucinations retrochiasmatiques. *Schweiz Med Wochenschr.* 1936;66: 700–8.
21. de Morsier G, Le Syndrome de Charles Bonnet: Hallucinations visuelles des vieillards sans déficience mentale. *Ann Méd Psychol.* 1967;125: 677–702.
22. Menon GJ, et al., Complex visual hallucinations in the visually impaired: The Charles Bonnet Syndrome. *Surv Ophthalmol.* 2003;48: 58–72.
23. Claparède H, *La Psychologie Animale de Charles Bonnet (Mémoire Publié á l'Occasion du Jubilé de l'Université. 1559–1909).* Geneva: Georg; 1909: 21.
24. Levêque de Pouilly JS, *Éloge de Charles Bonnet.* Lausanne: Henbach; 1794: 120–1.
25. Hughes Mearns. 1899 *Antigonish.* Harvard University student work and from the play *Psycho-Ed (sic)* 1910.
26. Lebel S, et al., *PLoS One.* 2020. https://doi.org/10.1371/journal.pone.0234124.
27. O'Brien J, et al., Visual hallucinations in neurological and ophthalmological disease: pathophysiology and management. *J Neurol Neurosurg Psychiatry.* 2020;5: 512–9.
28. Jones L, et al. Sometimes the whole room morphs into a different place. *Br Psychol Soc, The Psychologist.* 2021. https://www.bps.org.uk/psychologist/sometimes-whole-room-morphs-different-place.
29. Kaanders P, et al. Humans actively sample evidence to support prior beliefs *elife.* 2022. https://doi.org/10.7554/eLife.81228.
30. Fisher P, et al., *Routledge.* 2009. https://doi.org/10.4324/9780203881477.
31. Jones L, et al. From research to action: recommendations for Charles Bonnet syndrome care and policy. *BMJ Open Ophthalmol* 2025;10:e002009. https://doi.org/10.1136/bmjophth-2024-002009. https://bmjophth.bmj.com/content/bmjophth/10/1/e002009.full.pdf.
32. Hanoglu T, et al., Resting-state neural networks at complex visual hallucinations in Charles Bonnet Syndrome. *Authorea.* 2023; [online preprint] [accessed 6/12/2025].
33. Montagnese M, et al., A review of multimodal hallucinations: Categorization, assessment, theoretical perspectives, and clinical recommendations. *Schizophr Bull.* 2021;47(1): 237–48.
34. Kukstas C, Auditory Charles Bonnet syndrome: case report. *Br J Gen Pract.* 2019;69(684): 362–3.
35. Moreno Menguiano C, et al., What we know about Auditory Charles Bonnet Syndrome? *Eur Psych.* 2022; https://doi.org/10.1192/j.eurpsy.2022.1682 [accessed 7/16/2025].
36. Martínez Piera O, et al., Auditory Charles Bonnet syndrome and psychosis: Is there a relation? – A case report. *Psych Res Case Reports.* 2023;2(3): Article 100172. https://doi.org/10.1016/j.psycr.2023.100172. [accessed 7/16/2025].

37. *Vision & Eye Health Surveillance System (VEHSS)*, Centers for Disease Control and Prevention, Vision Health Initiative. [online] [accessed 6/12/2025].
38. Personal communication: Peter Ginsberg, Foundation Fighting Blindness, 6/11/2025.

Chapter 2

NEGATIVE VISUAL PHENOMENA

Smaran Teru and Leonid Skorin, Jr.

Introduction

> "Ти насправді не бачиш світ, якщо дивишся лише через своє власне вікно"
>
> "You don't really see the world if you only look through your own window."
>
> **—Ukrainian proverb**

Before we can understand positive visual phenomena such as illusions and visual hallucinations, one needs to address their antithesis, negative visual phenomena. These visual deficits can originate from the eye itself or anywhere along the visual pathway as it extends from the globe to the occipital lobe. This absence of visual information can present as visual acuity (VA) loss, scotomas in the field of vision, a myriad of visual field defects, or as visual distortion when a person perceives a typically normal image as broken, fractured, or even underwater.

Measuring Visual Acuity

Assessing negative visual phenomena begins with an ocular physical examination by first evaluating a patient's VA in each eye. VA is a measure of the eyes' ability to discern detailed visual stimuli and is often assessed with printed or projected letters or symbols known as optotypes.[1] Assessing distance and near VA evaluates the entire functional visual pathway as light passes through the anterior to posterior segment structures before being converted into electrical signals processed by the brain.[2] Measuring distance VA is the first step when evaluating your patient. It is important to note, however, that a chemical eye injury is the only ocular emergency in which VA assessment should be deferred to allow for immediate treatment. This consists of prompt administration of a topical anesthetic (and potentially an eyelid speculum or Morgan Lens in severe cases where the eye cannot be opened despite analgesia) and irrigation for a minimum of 30 minutes, followed by assessment of ocular pH.[3] In non-emergent situations, have the patient seated comfortably 6 meters (20 feet) from the VA chart with ample room light. For patients who are bedridden, or patients examined in the emergency room, proceed to the section below outlining near VA assessment. In smaller room spaces, mirrors are often used to achieve the required distance for accurate assessment.[4] The goal of measuring VA is to

DOI: 10.1201/9781003633365-2

determine a patient's monocular best-corrected visual acuity (BCVA). Doing so allows clinicians to evaluate for unilateral visual defects that may be masked if one does a binocular vision assessment alone.

It is preferable to test VA without correction first and then measure it again using the patient's most current spectacle or contact lens correction. Ask the patient to cover their left eye without pressing on it, preferably using an ophthalmic eye occluder; alternatively, a card, hand, or tissue can suffice if an occluder is unavailable.[1] Using a Snellen VA chart, ask the patient to read from left to right the top line of the chart and continue to the smallest line they can interpret. VA is listed as a Snellen fraction with the numerator indicating the patient's distance from the chart, and the denominator indicating the distance at which a normal eye can read that line of the chart.[1] For example, a VA of 6/24 (20/80) indicates that what the patient sees at 6 meters (20 feet) is equivalent to what a normal eye can see at 24 meters (80 feet). The uppermost (or largest) letter typically equates to a Snellen fraction of 6/60 (20/200).[5] For patients unable to read the largest Snellen optotype at 6 meters (20 feet) in either eye, move them closer to the Snellen chart and reassess.[1] For example, if a patient can read the uppermost letter at 3 meters (10 feet), the VA should be recorded as 3/60 (10/200). For patients unable to read the Snellen chart at any distance, reassess by holding up any number of fingers at 1 meter (3 feet), and ask whether they can accurately count them.[1] If they can, their VA is recorded as counting fingers (CF). For patients unable to count fingers, wave your hand first vertically, then horizontally at a closer distance to assess for hand motion, and ask whether they can accurately describe the direction of hand movement.[1] If they can, their VA is recorded as hand motion (HM). For patients unable to see hand motion, dim the room lights and shine a light toward the eye from various directions at an even closer distance, and ask whether they can see where the light is coming from.[1] If they can, their VA is recorded as light projection (LProject). If the patient cannot see from which direction the light is emanating, but can see whether the light is on or off, this is recorded as light perception (LPercept). If the patient cannot distinguish any light, they have no light perception (NLP). For unresponsive or comatose patients, a thorough pupillary examination should be performed, as described further below. After recording vision in the right eye, measure vision in the left eye, proceeding with the same steps outlined above.

After recording the patient's VA in both eyes separately without and with their habitual correction (spectacles, contact lenses), repeat the same steps using the pinhole eye occluder to identify possible improvements in their vision in each eye (Figure 2.1). Normally, peripheral and central light rays from a distant object are refracted (or bent) by the cornea and lens onto a specific point on the retina. In certain instances, light will focus in front of the retina, behind the retina, or at multiple points on the retina, producing a blurred image.[6] The pinhole occluder functions as a tiny aperture, selectively allowing central light

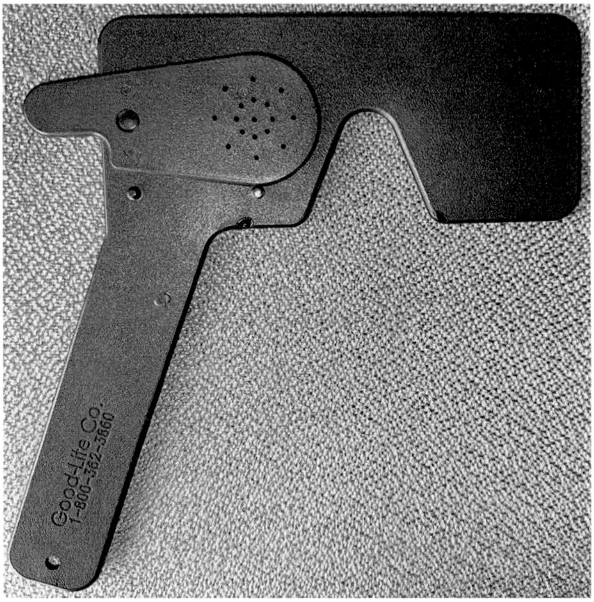

Figure 2.1 Pinhole occluder.

rays to enter. Because these central rays enter nearly perpendicular to the cornea, they do not require significant refraction and focus closer to the fovea on the retina, producing a sharper image.[6] Therefore, improvement in vision with pinhole testing suggests that the blurred vision is primarily due to a refractive error, as the eye is unable to adequately focus light onto the retina.

For patients evaluated outside the clinic, VA can still be measured using the same processes outlined earlier, but with a printed hand card (Rosenbaum pocket vision screener, Lebensohn chart, etc.) held 40 cm (16 inches) away with ample room lighting (Figure 2.2).[7] The printed hand card will often include a distance equivalent, noted as a Snellen fraction.

After thoroughly completing distance BCVA, proceed with near VA assessment. Near VA assesses the patient's vision at a normal reading distance. As we age, our natural lens loses elasticity and can no longer change shape to focus on near objects, a process known as presbyopia.[8] Patients, therefore, often wear glasses that add power, using a plus or convex lens (bifocal), to bring near target objects into focus. If applicable, instruct the patient to wear their reading glasses and follow the occlusion steps above for monocular VA evaluation. Instances where a patient's reading glasses are outdated, a phoropter or a manual trial lens set may be required to adjust the lens power and identify the appropriate near refraction.[7] Record the patient's near BCVA using the Jaeger notation or Snellen fraction found on the handheld chart. Among the various VA charts available, the Snellen chart is the most commonly used for adults who are familiar with the Roman alphabet.[9] For illiterate or non-English-speaking patients, the

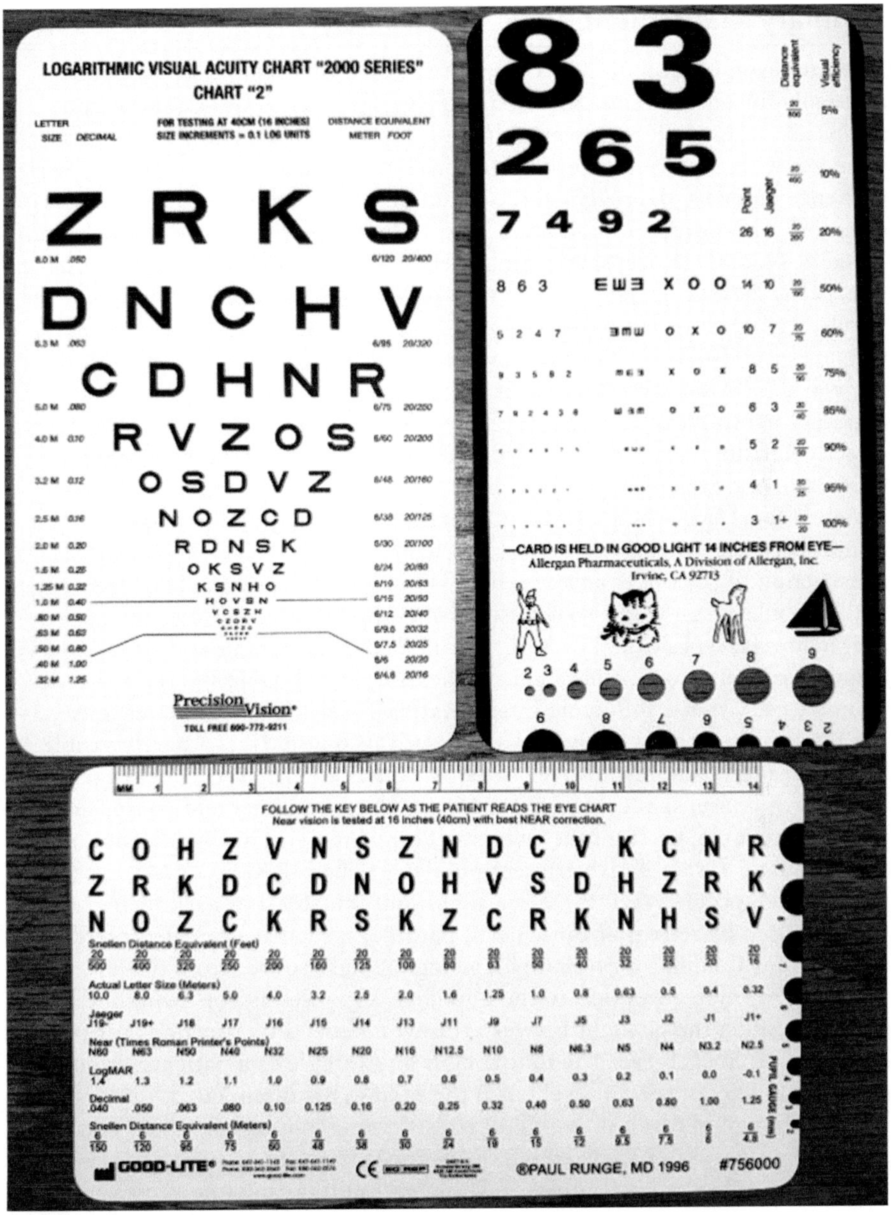

Figure 2.2 Various near-point eye charts.

Landolt C or Illiterate E charts are often used, where geometrically consistent configurations of letters C and E are displayed, and patients are asked to communicate which direction they point.[9] For children, LEA Symbols and Allen charts are often used, featuring photographic optotypes of familiar symbols and objects.[5, 10]

Pupillary Assessment

Pupillary examination is a key component of the ophthalmic workup, but especially for unresponsive or comatose patients, where subjective VA cannot be ascertained. Pupillary examination begins with measuring pupillary diameter with a measurement tool (often found on a near-point VA card with reference pupillary diameters graded in millimeters). Begin your assessment in the room with normal illumination, noting the diameter of both pupils in millimeters. Note their size, shape, and orientation as they should appear equal in size, perfectly round, and centered within the iris.[11] Compare the size of both pupils, paying close attention to anisocoria, or unequal pupil sizes. Normal physiological differences in pupil diameter affect approximately 20% of the population.[12] After recording pupil sizes, check for direct and consensual pupillary light reflexes. Ask the patient to fixate on a distant part of the room directly in front of their line of vision. Using a transilluminator or penlight, illuminate one eye, approaching it from a 30° angle at 1/3 meters (approximately 1 foot) from the patient.[11] Observe for prompt pupillary constriction in both the eye directly exposed to light and the opposite eye. Pupillary constriction of the eye exposed to light is known as the direct light reflex, while pupillary constriction of the opposite pupil is referred to as the consensual light reflex. In normal eyes, direct and consensual pupillary responses are equal. Direct and consensual light reflexes are graded subjectively on a scale from 0 to 4 with the following interpretation: 4+ is a brisk, large response, 3+ is a moderate response, 2+ is a small, slowed response, 1+ is a barely visible response, and 0 is unresponsive.[13] Pay particular attention to any differences in direct or consensual constriction. After evaluating direct and consensual pupillary reflexes, perform the swinging flashlight test. This pupil examination evaluates for a relative afferent pupillary deficit (RAPD) or Marcus Gunn pupil, which occurs when there is a significant unilateral or asymmetric visual defect caused by retinal or optic nerve pathology, such as optic neuropathy.[14] With a transilluminator or penlight, swing the light source from one eye to the next. Pay close attention to the pupillary responses as you swing the light. When swinging the penlight between the eyes, allow 3 to 5 seconds for pupillary reaction in each eye. The following is an example of a patient with optic nerve pathology of the left eye: when the right eye is illuminated (direct reflex), the left eye would result in pupillary constriction (consensual reflex) equal to that of the right eye. As you swing the penlight from the right eye to the left eye, both pupils would paradoxically dilate, resulting from the decreased light perception in the left eye because of the optic nerve damage.[8, 14] The RAPD can be graded subjectively on a scale from 0 to 4 or, for more accuracy, objectively using neutral density filters.[14]

Factors Affecting Visual Acuity

Normal vision (emmetropia) features light that focuses sharply on the retina without the need for optical or surgical refractive correction.[7] However, several important characteristics of the eye can result in the absence of emmetropia, also known as ametropia, where light is unable to focus directly on the retina.[7]

Ametropia can be classified as axial or refractive in etiology, encompassing conditions such as myopia, hyperopia, and astigmatism. The axial length of the eye may be increased (such as in myopia) or decreased (such as in hyperopia).[6] In myopic eyes, light rays focus anterior to the retina due to excessive convergent power, which refers to how strongly the eye refracts incoming light onto a focus point. This can occur as a result of increased corneal steepness or increased relative eye length.[7] In hyperopic eyes, light rays focus posterior to the retina due to insufficient convergent power, resulting from corneal flattening or decreased relative eye length.[7] Myopia can be corrected with a divergent (minus or concave) lens and hyperopia is corrected with a convergent (plus or convex) lens.[7] Astigmatism refers to irregularities in the shape of the cornea or natural lens, causing light rays to focus on multiple focal points, resulting in blurry vision.[6]

In addition to refractive etiologies, contrast sensitivity can also influence VA. The visual system is both contrast-sensitive and light-sensitive. Contrast sensitivity refers to the ability to detect differences in relative darkness and brightness. Even with 6/6 (20/20) VA, patients can have impaired contrast sensitivity, manifesting as an inability to discern details, edges, or borders of images.[7] Evaluation of contrast sensitivity involves letter-based charts or grating-based tests. In letter-based charts such as the Pelli-Robson or Regan charts, large letters of uniform size but progressively decreasing contrast are displayed.[6] Patients will continue to read the letters until they can correctly identify the letters at the lowest contrast level. In grating-based charts, alternating light and dark bars vary in spatial frequency (referring to relative thickness) and contrast.[7] Patients are asked to identify the orientation of gratings (left-tilted, right-tilted, or vertical) until they can accurately orient the gratings at the lowest contrast level.[7]

In addition to contrast sensitivity, pupils can influence VA. Pupillary diameter controls the relative amount of light that can enter the posterior segment of the eye. A larger pupillary diameter will allow more light rays to be transmitted, particularly peripheral light rays. Peripheral light rays experience different amounts of refraction compared to central light rays through a process known as spherical aberration.[6] Peripheral light rays are refracted more and converge earlier, focusing light in front of the retina, similarly to that of a myopic eye.[6] This becomes clinically relevant as the pupils normally dilate in the dark, causing more refraction of peripheral light entry and producing halos, glare, and ghosting of vision that is worse in myopic patients. Spherical aberration is always a consideration in laser-refractive and cataract surgery to minimize post-operative vision complications. Furthermore, the Stiles-Crawford effect states that light entering through the center of the pupil is perceived as brighter and more effective than light entering near the edge, even when both have the same physical intensity.[15] Cone cells in the retina—most dense in the fovea—are angled toward the pupillary center and absorb more central light rays than those entering at an angle from the periphery.[15] In bright light, our pupils normally constrict to allow only central light rays, thereby producing sharper vision that projects to the fovea. Note that along with vision and pupils, a thorough ocular examination also includes assessments of intraocular pressure, extraocular motility, and confrontation visual fields (which will be discussed further below).

Visual Field Anatomy and Deficits

Understanding visual field deficits first requires an overview of the anatomical visual pathway. The concept of how objects in our visual field project to certain regions of the retina can be confusing, so here is an example. Imagine you are walking down the street, and you see a small red balloon floating in the upper left corner of your visual field. The light reflected from the balloon enters both eyes but is transmitted to the inferior nasal retina of the left eye and the inferior temporal retina of the right eye. The visual field and retina have an inverted and reversed relationship.[16] Relative to the fixation point, light from objects in the upper visual field falls on the inferior retina below the fovea, from the lower visual field on the superior retina above the fovea, light from the nasal visual field falls on the temporal retina, and from the temporal visual field falls on the nasal retina.[16] Therefore, where an object is in our visual field controls where on the retina it is transmitted. The optic nerve, which consists of approximately 1.1 million axons, transmits information from the retina to the brain along the visual pathway.[17] Optic nerve axons from the nasal retina of both eyes will eventually cross to the contralateral side via a bundle of nerve fibers known as the optic chiasm.[16] In our red balloon example, axons transmitting information from the nasal retina of the left eye will eventually cross in the optic chiasm and join the axons transmitting information from the temporal retina of the right eye (which do not cross in the chiasm) to create the right optic tract.[16] The optic tract will transmit this information to the lateral geniculate nucleus (LGN).[16] From the LGN, optic radiations transmit information to the visual cortex in the occipital region.[16] Optic radiations are often characterized by inferior and superior designations, based on the area of the retina stimulated.[16] Therefore, accurately interpreting visual field deficits requires a solid understanding of how specific regions of the retina correspond to areas of the visual field and how lesions along the visual pathway disrupt this mapping. An overview of the visual pathway is shown in Figure 2.3.

Confrontation visual fields, which are usually done during a comprehensive eye examination, are a quick method for assessing gross visual field deficits. Each eye is tested individually. Ask the patient to fixate on your nose from a distance of 1 meter (3 feet). Hold your hands midway between yourself and the patient in opposite quadrants, 20° and 30° from central fixation (24 inches from the mutual axis).[16] Display 1, 2, or 5 fingers in all four quadrants (superior temporal, superior nasal, inferior temporal, and inferior nasal) and note if the patient is unable to identify the number of fingers in these quadrants accurately.[16] If a field defect is detected, formal computerized visual field testing is warranted.

The Amsler grid is also a quick and non-invasive method to detect macular and paracentral visual field abnormalities, particularly in the central 20° of fixation.[8] The grid consists of 20 rows and 20 columns, forming 400 individual 5-mm squares.[8] It features evenly spaced horizontal and vertical black lines on a white background, with a small central black dot for fixation (Figure 2.4).[8]

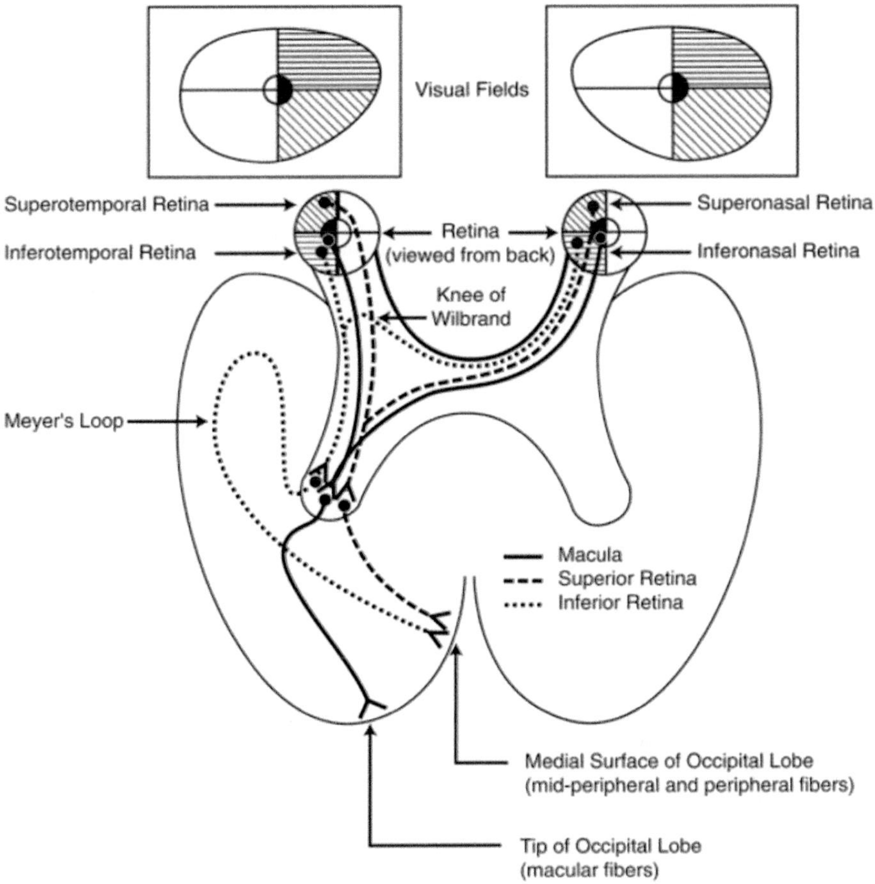

Figure 2.3 Anatomy of the visual pathway, beginning with light projected onto the nasal and temporal retina and ending with projections to the primary visual cortex. Courtesy of Foroozan R, Vaphiades MS, Visual fields. In: Foroozan R, Vaphiades MS, eds., *Klines Neuro-Ophthalmology Review Manual*, 8th edn. Boca Raton: Taylor & Francis; 2017: 16–31.

To use the Amsler grid, ask the patient to cover one eye. With the chart well illuminated at a comfortable reading distance, ask the patient to look directly at the central dot and maintain this fixation throughout the entire exam. Then, ask the patient to report any distortion or waviness of the lines on the grid. Also, ask if the patient can see all four outside corners of the grid and all four sides of the square. Repeat testing in the other eye. Distortion or wavy appearance of the lines on the Amsler grid is known as metamorphopsia, which is highly suggestive of macular pathology, such as age-related macular degeneration, macular edema, central serous chorioretinopathy, epiretinal membrane, etc.[7] A missing central dot or lines on the Amsler grid is concerning for a central, cecocentral, or paracentral scotoma which can present with a macular hole (Figure 2.5).[8]

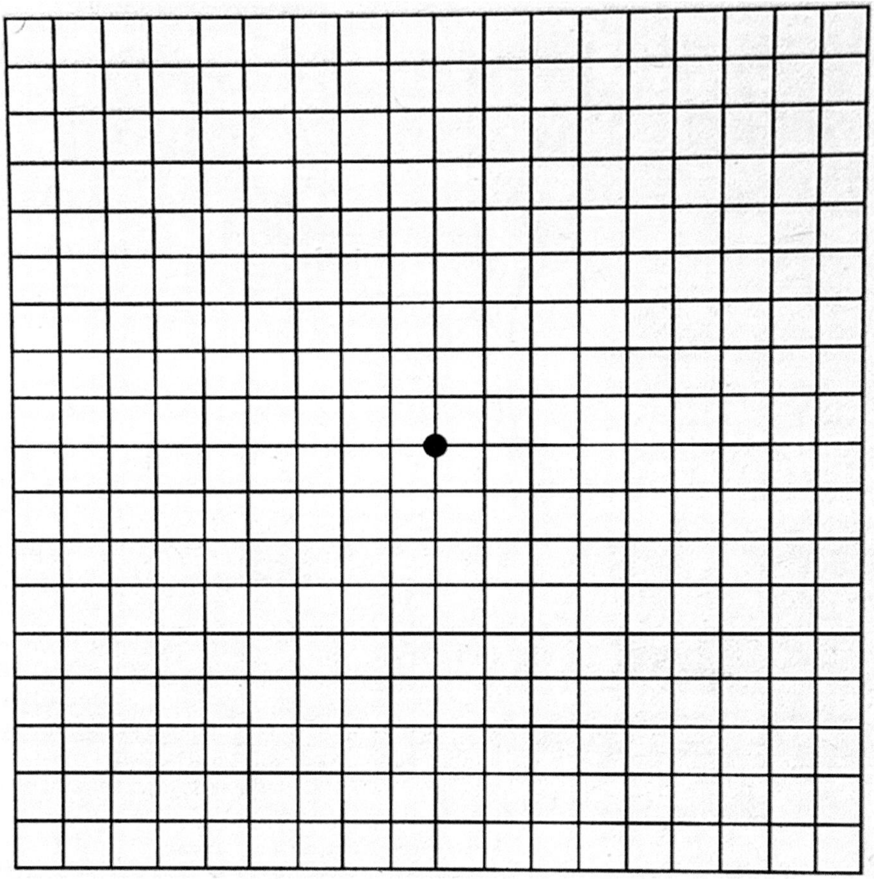

Figure 2.4 Amsler grid.

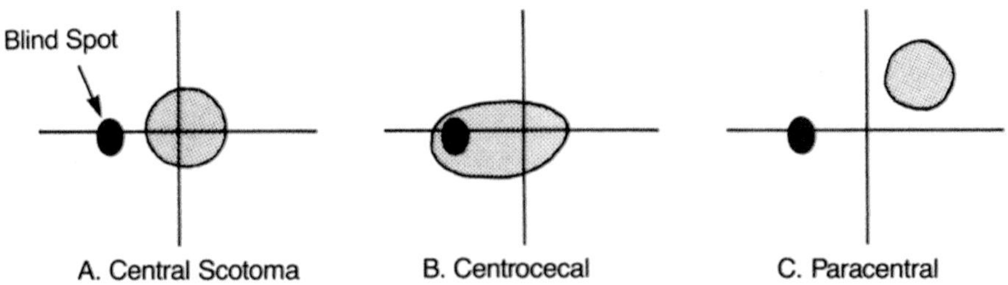

Figure 2.5 Visual demonstration of central, cecocentral (encompassing the fixation point and blind spot), and paracentral (outside the point of fixation and not involving the blind spot) scotomas involving lesions at the papillomacular bundle. The center at both intersecting lines demarcates central fixation, and the gray figure demonstrates the scotoma. Courtesy Foroozan R, Vaphiades MS, Visual fields. In: Foroozan R, Vaphiades MS, eds., *Klines Neuro-Ophthalmology Review Manual*, 8th edn. Boca Raton: Taylor & Francis; 2017: 16-31.

Patients can perform Amsler grid testing at home to help monitor subjective progression of macular function.

Anterior to Posterior Segment Pathology Affecting Visual Acuity

Understanding how different pathologies in the visual pathway can affect VA requires a systematic approach from the anterior to the posterior segments. Inadequate tear volume or function can result in a dry or inflamed ocular surface. Tear film abnormalities can manifest as ocular surface disease that can cause light scattering or blurry vision. The cornea is a complex structure that is responsible for approximately 75% of the eye's optical power.[8] Irregularities in corneal shape, such as astigmatism, keratoconus, postsurgical ectasia, corneal scarring from infection or trauma, and edema, as seen in bullous keratopathy or Fuchs' dystrophy, can all impact normal corneal refractive function and power, affecting both its transparency and shape.[17] Between the cornea and the iris is the anterior chamber, filled with aqueous humor.[7] Accumulation of blood (hyphema) or white blood cells (hypopyon) in the anterior chamber can obscure the visual axis and prevent light from reaching the retina in severe instances. Hyphemas most commonly result from blunt force trauma, tearing fragile iris and ciliary body blood vessels.[8] Other etiologies include iris neovascularization from poorly controlled diabetic retinopathy, retinal venous occlusion, blood dyscrasias such as sickle cell disease, or anticoagulation use.[8] Hyphemas are graded by severity and may require prompt surgical intervention depending on intraocular pressure and the nature of the injury.[7] The pupil is the central opening of the iris, and its size and reactivity depend on normal iris sphincter and dilator muscular functions. In bright light, the iris sphincter muscle normally contracts, causing pupillary constriction, while, in dim light, the iris sphincter muscle relaxes and the iris dilator muscle contracts, causing pupillary dilation.[8, 18] Pathologies involving the iris can therefore affect VA, including traumatic mydriasis, iridodialysis, and anterior or posterior synechia. In traumatic mydriasis, blunt force trauma damages the iris sphincter muscle and prevents iris contraction.[7] This, in turn, results in unopposed pupillary dilation, allowing more light to enter uncontrollably, causing glare, photophobia, and blurry vision. In iridodialysis, the iris is disinserted from the scleral spur, often preceded by blunt force trauma.[19] Depending on the size of iris disinsertion, glare, photophobia, and monocular diplopia may result. Damage to the trabecular meshwork can result in elevated intraocular pressure and peripheral anterior synechiae. Synechiae are fibrous adhesions between the iris and cornea (anterior) or between the iris and natural lens (posterior) that are often caused by inflammation.[7] Anterior or posterior synechiae that extend the entire circumference of the pupillary margin (also known as seclusion pupillae) obstruct aqueous flow from the posterior to the anterior chambers, causing the iris to bow anteriorly from the increased pressure in the posterior chamber. This process is implicated in acute angle-closure glaucoma, an ophthalmic emergency with potentially catastrophic visual outcomes. As previously discussed, pathologic or physiologic differences in pupillary diameter can influence the relative amount of light entering the eye, affecting depth of focus and image quality. A cataract is when the natural lens opacifies and can result from aging, systemic disease, or trauma.[8] The cataract's effect on VA depends on the type, extent, and position of the opacification. Cataracts result in glare, blurry vision, poor night vision, color perception issues, and monocular diplopia.[8] Age-acquired cataracts are the most common and include nuclear sclerotic, cortical, and subcapsular cataracts, depending on the anatomic location of the opacification. Posterior to the lens lies the vitreous, a clear gel-like substance that fills the space between the lens and retina. It maintains the ocular shape, provides a clear medium for light to reach the retina, and acts as a shock absorber in the eye.[20] Vitreous hemorrhage, inflammatory debris, and opacities can affect VA. Posterior to the vitreous lies the retina, a thin-layered sheet of neural tissue that functions to convert light into electrical signals for central interpretation and processing by the visual cortex of the brain.[21] The retina consists of photoreceptor cells (rods and cones) for light detection and neuronal cells (including bipolar and ganglion cell types) for central transmission. Key portions of the retina include the macula, a small oval-shaped and cone-dense region of the central retina, and the fovea, a pit-like depression in the central macula that contains the highest concentration of cones.[20] Vascular (diabetic retinopathy, hypertensive retinopathy, retinal artery/vein occlusion, etc.) or structural (retinal detachment, macular holes, central serous retinopathy, macular degeneration, etc.) pathologies within the retina can also affect VA. Damage to the optic nerve, as seen in glaucoma, optic neuritis (such as in infections or autoimmune diseases), or ischemic optic neuropathy, affects the transmission of visual information. Finally, lesions to the visual pathway caused by tumors, trauma, or ischemic infarct that involve the optic tract, radiations, or visual cortex can produce variable VA effects involving all or part of the patients' vision. As a result, structural or functional aberration to any part of the visual system will affect the patient's ultimate visual performance.

Illustrative Case

A 34-year-old male was seen in the eye clinic after first presenting to the emergency department (ED) earlier that same day. He stated that half of his vision had disappeared suddenly, eleven hours before his ED visit. He also complained of a pounding headache located at the back of his head. It started at the same time as his vision loss and had been getting progressively worse. Other positive symptoms included nausea and photophobia. He denied dizziness, numbness, tingling, or weakness. The patient stated that he was in good physical health and denied any head injuries or illnesses. The patient had a history of migraine headaches but was not prescribed medications for them. He was on an albuterol inhaler, as needed, for asthma. The patient was taking clonazepam and nortriptyline for depression. He had one episode of "stroke" four years earlier, where he developed left-sided weakness, short-term memory loss, and stuttering. He did not recall any work-up or neuroimaging during that event. All those symptoms were resolved after rehabilitation therapy. The patient smoked one pack of cigarettes per day for 20 years. He denied any recent alcohol or illicit drug use.

In the ED, his blood pressure was 149 mmHg/85 mmHg. All additional testing, including a complete blood count with differential, basic metabolic panel, and computed tomography of the head without contrast, was unremarkable. The patient had mild myopia in both eyes, corrected with habitual glasses to 20/20 right eye, 20/20 left eye, and 20/15 both eyes at distance. The pupil responses were normal; there was no afferent pupillary defect. Extraocular muscle testing was remarkable for excessive refixations. He did not exhibit nystagmus. Formal computerized visual field testing identified a left homonymous hemianopia (Figure 2.6a and b). Due to this visual field defect finding, the patient was referred to the neurology stroke service. On magnetic resonance imaging of the brain, the patient was found to have infarcts predominantly involving the right occipital lobe (Figure 2.7). No definitive etiology for his stroke was ever established. The patient was told to start 81 mg of aspirin and 75 mg of clopidogrel and was to continue his other regular medications.

The patient was seen again in the eye clinic a couple weeks after his initial visit. His ocular evaluation was unchanged. He stated that he was trying to quit smoking by using nicotine replacement therapy. At that visit, the patient was counseled regarding his homonymous hemianopia. The reported rate of spontaneous improvement of blind hemifields in patients with homonymous hemianopia varies between 18% and 67% but recovery is negligible after two to three

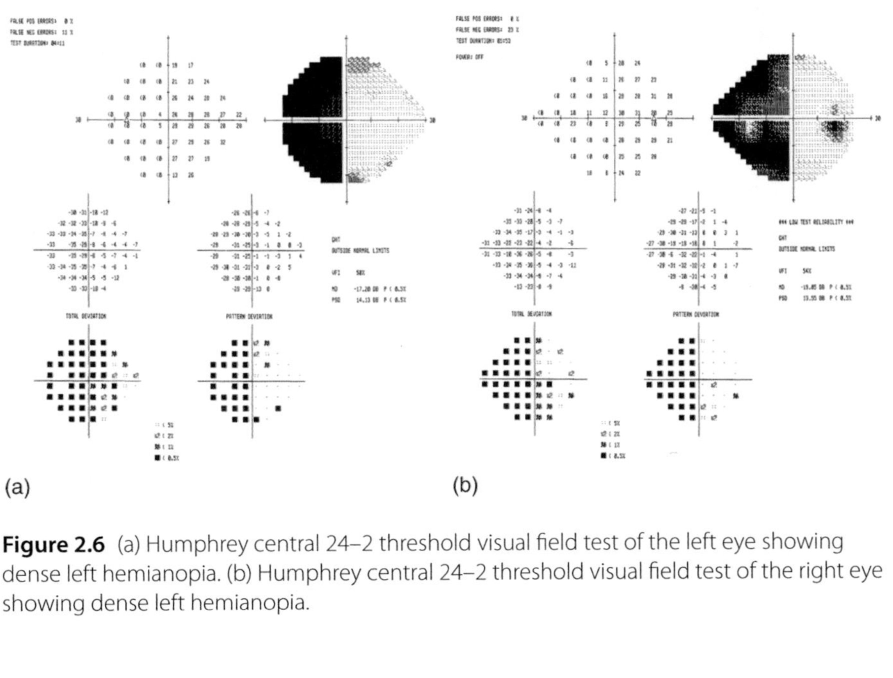

(a) (b)

Figure 2.6 (a) Humphrey central 24–2 threshold visual field test of the left eye showing dense left hemianopia. (b) Humphrey central 24–2 threshold visual field test of the right eye showing dense left hemianopia.

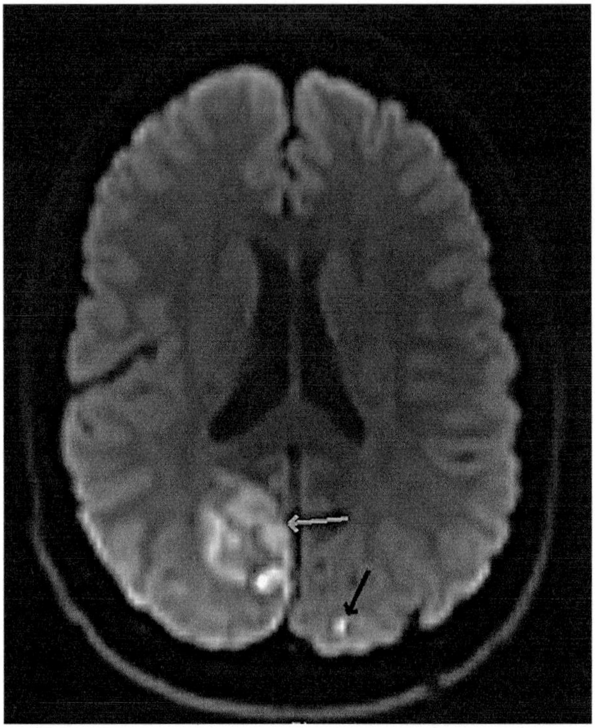

Figure 2.7 Axial diffusion weighted imaging. Magnetic resonance imaging showing large area of infarction in the right occipital lobe (white arrow) and a smaller focal area of infarction at the tip of the left occipital lobe (black arrow).

months and unlikely after six months.[21, 22] Visual field defects that result from a vascular etiology, such as in this patient, are the least likely to show improvement.[21, 22] If improvement does occur, it is seen in stages starting with perception of light, motion, form, color, and finally depth.[21, 22]

Optical devices and aids are the most frequently utilized treatment modality for patients with homonymous hemianopia (see Chapter 9).[21, 23] The patient needs to be highly motivated and must practice with the device. Many patients are confused by the optics of these systems and can feel nauseated while wearing them. The goal is to help patients increase their ability to successfully complete their activities of daily living. After appropriate adaptation, these devices can improve ambulation but generally may not be used for driving. Some newer prism placement modalities may now give patients the ability to drive in some locations.[24] The optical device that was trialed for our patient was placement of bilateral yoked prisms. Yoked prisms, whether added unilaterally or bilaterally to a spectacle correction, shifts any images from the blind field into the seeing field. This essentially shifts the location of the field and is not a true expansion of the field. The prescription of bilateral yoked prisms can result in reduced visual acuities due to decreased image quality. Ten prism diopters base left before each eye was trialed on our patient. With this prism, the patient reported being able to see the doors on his left as he walked down the hallway in the eye clinic. He did not notice that his right visual field was any smaller. This prism arrangement did make him slightly nauseated. Since this was relatively early after his stroke and vision loss event, the patient decided against trying the prism at this time and instead waited for possible recovery or adaptation to his vision loss. Future intervention depends upon the patient's needs, activities, and specific deficits. Many variables can be altered to allow significant improvement in their quality of life and help them focus on making the most of their remaining vision.

REFERENCES

1. Marsden J, et al., How to measure distance visual acuity. *Community Eye Health*. 2014;27(85):16.
2. Mahabadi N, et al., Neuroanatomy, Retina. In: *StatPearls*. Treasure Island (FL): StatPearls Publishing; August 8, 2023.
3. Fish R, et al., Management of ocular thermal and chemical injuries, including amniotic membrane therapy. *Curr Opin Ophthalmol.* 2010;21(4):317–21.
4. Daiber HF, et al., Visual Acuity. In: *StatPearls*. Treasure Island (FL): StatPearls Publishing; May 29, 2023.
5. Caltrider D, et al., Evaluation of visual acuity. In: *StatPearls*. Treasure Island (FL): StatPearls Publishing; May 1, 2024.
6. Brodie SE, et al., eds., *Clinical Optics and Vision Rehabilitation*, 10th edn. San Francisco, CA: American Academy of Ophthalmology; 2025: 88–89, 143–166.
7. Blomquist OH, ed., *Practical Ophthalmology: A Manual for Beginner Residents*, 8th edn. San Francisco, CA: American Academy of Ophthalmology; 2025: 27–31, 39, 47–55, 295.
8. Salmon JF, *Kanski's Clinical Ophthalmology: A Systematic Approach*, 10th edn. Elsevier; 2025: 5–6, 206, 308–313, 390, 395, 731.
9. Azzam D, et al., Snellen chart. In: *StatPearls*. Treasure Island (FL): StatPearls Publishing; May 1, 2023.
10. Vivekanand U, et al., Is LEA symbol better compared to Snellen chart for visual acuity assessment in preschool children? *Rom J Ophthalmol.* 2019;63(1):35–7.
11. Biller J, et al., Examination of the peripheral ocular motor system. In: *DeMyer's The Neurologic Examination: A Programmed Text*, 7th edn. Philadelphia, PA: McGraw-Hill; 2016: 151–155.
12. Lam BL, et al., The prevalence of simple anisocoria. *Am J Ophthalmol.* 1987;104(1):69–73.
13. Belliveau AP, et al., Pupillary light reflex. In: *StatPearls*. Treasure Island (FL): StatPearls Publishing; July 25, 2023.

14. Skorin L, et al., Pupil abnormalities. In: Onofrey BE, Skorin L, Holdeman NR, eds., *Ocular Therapeutics Handbook: A Clinical Manual*, 4th edn. Philadelphia: Wolters Kluwer; 2020: 578–80.
15. Snyder AW, et al., The Stiles–Crawford effect – explanation and consequences. *Vision Res.* 1973;13(6):1115–37.
16. Foroozan R, et al., Visual fields. In: Foroozan R, Vaphiades MS, eds., *Kline's Neuro-Ophthalmology Review Manual*, 8th edn. Boca Raton: Taylor & Francis; 2017: 16–31.
17. Trief D, et al., eds., *External Disease and Cornea*, 10th edn. San Francisco, CA: American Academy of Ophthalmology; 2025: 8–17, 99, 210–212, 217.
18. Bron AJ, et al., *Wolff's Anatomy of the Eye and Orbit*, 8th edn. London: Chapman & Hall Medical; 1997: 655–7.
19. Gervasio K, et al., *The Wills Eye Manual: Office and Emergency Room Diagnosis and Treatment of Eye Diseases*, 8th edn. Philadelphia, PA: Wolters Kluwer; 2021: Chapter 3: Trauma.
20. Kim SJ, et al., eds., *Retina and Vitreous*, 10th edn. San Francisco, CA: American Academy of Ophthalmology; 2025: 5, 7–15.
21. Pambakian AL, et al., *Br J Ophthalmol.* 1997. https://doi.org/10.1136/bjo.81.4.324
22. Zhang X, et al., Natural history of homonymous hemianopia. *Neurology.* 2006;66(6):901–5.
23. Biousse V, Newman N, *Neuro-Ophthalmology Illustrated*, 1st edn. New York: Thieme; 2009: 498–500.
24. Moss AM, et al., Patients with homonymous hemianopia become visually qualified to drive using novel monocular sector prisms. *J Neuroophthalmol.* 2014;34(1):53–6.

Chapter 3

POSITIVE VISUAL PHENOMENA

Gregory Gosdigian and Leonid Skorin, Jr.

Introduction

"Очі бачать далеко, але розум ще далі"

"The eyes see far, but the mind even further"

—Ukrainian proverb

Positive visual phenomena are defined as alterations in the size, shape, position, and motion of viewed objects. Common forms of these phenomena include flashing or flickering lights, various geometric shapes, and animated objects or scenes. People who have had strokes, migraines, or lesions in their brain are at a higher risk of developing these alterations. These phenomena are common in patients who have lesions that affect their ocular anatomy and visual pathways in the brain. Lesions within parts of the brain, optic radiations, and associated structures like the ophthalmic and maxillary branches of cranial nerve V, known as the trigeminal nerve, are noted to exhibit these changes.[1] Excitation to lesioned cortical parts of the brain occur within early visual areas. This leads to visual symptoms for at-risk individuals such as stroke patients. Patients who have migraines can also experience persistent positive visual events. In these situations, it is not uncommon to see simple or diffuse patterns that may resemble television static or dots running across the full visual field.[2]

Although we are aware of these visual alterations, it is important to distinguish them from each other to aid in the diagnostic process. The two groups of positive visual phenomena which patients can experience include illusions and hallucinations. To distinguish between them, illusions occur when viewed objects are misperceived, whereas hallucinations are visual experiences that occur due to internal neural activity rather than from an external source. Further separating them, hallucinations are perceptions in the absence of external stimuli, while illusions are the misinterpretations of actual stimuli present in the outside environment. When attempting to identify positive visual episodes, it is important to know that hallucinations can be formed images including specific objects and people, or unformed images such as light and geometric figures. This can originate from retinal or optic nerve lesions, seizures, migraines, visual pathway anomalies or even visual deprivation. On the other hand, illusions usually present as metamorphopsia, micropsia, macropsia, and palinopsia, which are typically found in patients with retinal, optic nerve, or cortical brain lesions.

DOI: 10.1201/9781003633365-3

Although both can be present in healthy patients, illusions are much more common in those suffering from epilepsy, migraine, or stroke.[3, 4]

Illusions

i. Misperceptions of viewed objects

Illusions are discrepancies between our perception and objective reality. For example, a patient complaining of visual experiences in only one eye can be experiencing a binocular hemifield phenomenon. This is because patients can often misinterpret a binocular hemifield phenomenon as a monocular phenomenon due to the difference in their perceptions and what is occurring. Patient cases like these often reveal certain limitations of the brain's processing capabilities of sensory information.[5]

ii. Mistaking a rope for a snake

One example of what patients might go through when experiencing an illusion is mistaking a rope as a snake. The fascinating thing about this is that research suggests this illusion is influenced by not only visual features, but also the context of the perception. Curvilinear shapes, including both ropes and snakes, are known to lead to enhanced electrophysiological responses. This happens particularly when snakes are expected in the context in which they are observed.[6] There is also the concept of the "Rotating Snakes" illusion in which a person can believe that static images are moving due to the activated motion-sensitive areas within the visual cortex of the human visual system, particularly during eye movements.[7] This phenomenon displays the connection between low-level visual processing and high-level cognitive features of illusory perception.

iii. Polka dots on a dress seen as insects

Another example of an illusion is observing polka dots on a dress and interpreting them as insects. This illusion also occurs due to the context of the perception such as the previous scenario of misinterpreting a rope for a snake. For example, if a person experiencing this illusion is outdoors, where insects are commonly found, it is more reasonable that someone wearing a polka dotted dress has bugs on them if the viewer is suffering from some form of vision loss.

Hallucinations

i. Sensory perception of things not there

Hallucinations are traditionally defined as the perception of sensory information in the absence of external stimuli. A potentially better definition in such circumstances, that provides more insight into what such hallucinations are, includes the unconstrained perceptions that arise from a decreased sensory input's impact on thalamocortical circuits. Ultimately, the hyperexcitability of the cortical brain, attentional mechanisms, and abnormal function of the thalamus can all contribute to the experience of hallucinations.[8] This prominent network plays a vital role in selecting sensory representations for human consciousness, but abnormal selection can often lead to hallucinations in schizophrenia spectrum disorders.[9]

ii. Subjective experience without objective stimuli

As previously stated, hallucinations are sensory perceptions that occur without external stimuli. This differentiates them from illusions which involve misinterpretation of actual stimuli. Hallucinations are associated with medical, neurological, and psychiatric conditions, but are also a part of normal human experience.[10] Recent studies show that initial prominent ideologies and beliefs play a vital role in the development of hallucinations, challenging earlier explanations that focused on internal cognitive disruptions.[11] Furthermore, neuroimaging research has explored the involvement of specific neurotransmitters and brain regions in hallucination generation, leading to the development of integrative models for hallucination production.[12]

iii. Persist with eye closure

One way to tell if a patient is experiencing a hallucination rather than an illusion is the persistence of sensory perception during eye closure. It has been documented that patients can experience visual hallucinations during eye closure in various conditions. Medically originated examples of these closed-eye conditions include atropine toxicity cases, severe withdrawal from alcohol, and hyponatremia.[13, 14] These types of hallucinations are usually vivid, full of color, and lifelike with patients often being aware of this phenomenon apart from their reality.[15] The time, detail, and transparency of experiences can also differ based on the specific eye closure condition a patient presents with.[16]

Pseudohallucinations

Pseudohallucinations are sensory experiences that are recognized by patients as not being real. This very concept distinguishes them from true hallucinations (see Chapter 7).[17] Certain cases where patients might experience this visual phenomenon include post-cardiac surgery and in instances of an uncommon neurological condition known as superficial siderosis.[18, 19] It is important to also note that the intensity of suicidal ideation is higher in patients experiencing pseudohallucinations when compared to both true hallucinations and no hallucinations in emergency psychiatric patients.[20]

As previously discussed in Chapter 1, the term pseudohallucination (with the above noted exceptions) is a rather confusing term, especially if it is applied to Charles Bonnet Syndrome (CBS). CBS is completely reviewed in Chapter 8. A brief introduction to CBS is warranted here. CBS is also known as a visual release phenomenon, which results in visual hallucinations in visually impaired individuals. It occurs more frequently, although not exclusively, in elderly patients who for the most part interpret their visual hallucinations as not being real.[21] In this condition, hallucinations are entirely visual, usually temporary, but may last for months or even years and often found in patients without any underlying mental or behavioral disorders. Despite its prevalence, CBS is often missed as a diagnosis, underdiagnosed or even misinterpreted as psychosis.[22]

As can be seen, making the correct diagnosis of CBS is difficult enough to do clinically without adding confusing concepts and terminology to the mix. In general terms, it is possible to apply both current sub-categories of pseudohallucinations to CBS. These include the patient experiencing a "hallucination with insight" into it not being real and the "vivid internal imagery".[23] A true visual hallucination is experienced as objective and located in external space which is what most CBS patients will tell us they perceive.[24]

As one can see from these definitions, CBS visual phenomena actually have key elements of both pseudohallucinations and true hallucinations. These would include being located in the external space either occupying the whole visualized space or superimposed upon a portion of the real scene behind or around the hallucinatory imagery. CBS patients know the images they see are not real. These images also usually have great vividness and clarity of the imaginary scene. At this time, no consistent operational definition has emerged for the term pseudohallucination.[17] The utility of the differentiation between true hallucinations and pseudohallucinations has been questioned and even rejected by various authors.[23, 25] The term pseudohallucination as it has been applied to CBS in the past is both confusing and inappropriate and therefore should no longer be used.

Both Types of Positive Visual Phenomena Occur from Disturbances of the Neural Visual Pathway

Both types of positive visual phenomena emanate from disturbances of the neural visual pathway. The difference lies in the fact that illusions may also be caused by optical abnormalities, whereas hallucinations are always neural events.[26] Visual perceptual abnormalities, including hallucinations and illusions, are complex phenomena that occur in many different neurological and psychiatric conditions. These distinctions are very important in the fields of psychiatry and psychology for descriptive purposes and neurology for understanding the mechanisms of neural networks. Various psychiatric conditions, such as mania and schizophrenia, can induce visual perceptual abnormalities, and different neurological disorders such as epilepsy, dementia, and stroke also have that ability.[27] Understanding the diverse causes and manifestations of these phenomena is crucial for accurate diagnosis and appropriate treatment.

In cases where visual hallucinations arise from psychiatric conditions, alcohol abuse or withdrawal, and drugs such as lysergic acid diethylamide and marijuana, these visual hallucinations can be very complex and have other accompanying sensory hallucinations. Visual phenomena reported by patients require comprehensive evaluation beyond self-description. A full neuro-ophthalmological examination, including visual acuity testing, visual field evaluation and complete external ocular and internal fundus examination, is necessary to determine the etiologies.[28]

Research suggests that hypertension may affect visual function even in the absence of eye disease. Studies have also found delayed visual evoked potential latencies in some hypertensive patients that point towards potential optic nerve involvement.[29] Additionally, hypertensive patients have been shown to have slightly reduced sensitivity loss to increased background illuminance and a potentially higher age-related rate of sensitivity loss for certain visual measures.[30] Interestingly, among normotensive individuals, cardiovascular factors such as blood pressure and heart rate were also connected with the suppression of long-wavelength-sensitive cone flicker responses.[30] These findings suggest that hypertension, or its treatment, may subtly impact visual function through various mechanisms, including vascular changes and potential demyelination in visual pathways.

Positive visual symptoms may be accompanied by occipital lobe seizures. Findings on electroencephalogram and magnetic resonance imaging may show transient abnormalities in the occipital lobe areas. Notably, these visual phenomena typically resolve with proper blood glucose control, often without the need for long-term antiepileptic medication.[31, 32] The recognition of hyperglycemia-induced visual disturbances is crucial for prompt diagnosis and treatment, as these symptoms can be mistaken for other neurological conditions. Ultimately, early intervention with insulin and rehydration is a major contributor to symptom resolution in these patients.[33]

Illusions—May Also be Caused by Optical Abnormalities

The optical disorders that generate illusions include improper refraction (causing altered shape) and cataractous or dislocated lenses (causing multiple images and altered color).[26] There are also retinal metamorphopsia, retinal macropsia and retinal micropsia which involve distortions or illusions that are caused by macular disease and displacement or scarring of the foveal cones.

It is important to note that diseases such as diabetes can lead to various visual phenomena and abnormal ocular changes. Diabetes can lead to degradation of retinal image quality due to increased ocular aberrations and scattering, and this primarily affects the tear film, cornea, and natural crystalline lens. Some diabetic individuals can even visualize their own parafoveal retinopathy with many being able to obtain an idea of their foveal avascular zone size.[34, 35]

Dense and bilateral cataracts have also been documented to induce visual phenomena as these are caused by optical abnormalities within the lens that can lead to illusions. Treatment options for illusions caused by these cataracts include phacoemulsification cataract surgery with intraocular lens implantation as this has been proven to be curative.[36] Abnormal visual acuity has also been associated with illusions, with no patients experiencing symptoms when visual acuity is normal. These findings suggest that addressing visual impairment through glasses, contact lenses or cataract surgery may be beneficial in managing or preventing illusions in affected patients.

Understanding and addressing these phenomena is crucial for improving patient satisfaction and surgical outcomes in cataract procedures. These phenomena provide insights into visual perception, aesthetics, and the neurological basis of visual experiences.

Hallucinations—Always Neural Events

Visual hallucinations originate from disorders of the retina, optic nerve, and areas of the brain related to vision including the occipital, parietal, or temporal cortex.[26] This supports our current understanding that hallucinations are without exception neural events that arise from complex brain processes. It has also been proposed that hallucinations derive from the inability to differentiate neural activity generated internally and externally, which is normally decoupled.[37]

In every case, monocular hallucinations always originate from abnormal functioning photoreceptors or optic nerves. This is important to appreciate because the nature of hallucinations provides us with an idea of their origin. Obtaining an enhanced understanding of these mechanisms may provide better insight into the neural basis of consciousness and potential therapeutic targets.[38]

Brain imaging and neurotransmission research have also shown how neurobiology and hallucinations are connected across various clinical conditions. It has even been argued that hallucinations are pathological not because they are self-generated by the patient, but because this self-generated neural activity is perceived as external.[24] Ultimately, these various perspectives conjointly support the concept that hallucinations are deeply embedded in neural processes and their misinterpretation.

Conclusion

A comprehensive eye exam is fundamental when trying to identify the underlying cause of a patient's positive visual phenomena. Clinicians should order supportive studies and consult with other specialists to rule out pertinent differentials and arrive at the appropriate diagnosis. This should be done before attributing a more benign diagnosis of exclusion to a patient's symptomatology. Finally, clinicians should strive to find the many potential underlying etiologies and other typical features of these conditions as they can help guide the doctor to the appropriate diagnosis and subsequent management.

REFERENCES

1. Baier B, et al., *Neurol.* 2010. https://doi.org/10.1212/WNL.0b013e3181cb3e64.
2. Liu GT, et al., *Neurol.* 1995. https://doi.org/10.1212/wnl.45.4.664.
3. Borruat FX, *Klin Monbl Augenheilkd.* 1999. https://doi.org/10.1055/s-2008-1034805.
4. Kölmel HW, Visual illusions and hallucinations. *Baillieres Clin Neurol.* 1993;2(2):243–264.
5. Bayne T, Perception and the reach of phenomenal content. *PQ.* 2009;59:385–404.
6. Grassini S, et al., *Emotion.* 2019. https://doi.org/10.1037/emo0000434.
7. Kuriki I, et al., *J Vis.* 2008. https://doi.org/10.1167/8.10.16.

8. Behrendt RP, et al., *Behav Brain Sci.* 2004. https://doi.org/10.1017/s0140525x04000184.
9. Hare SM, *Front Neurosci.* 2021. https://doi.org/10.3389/fnins.2021.733038.
10. Brasić JR, *Percept Mot Skills.* 1998. https://doi.org/10.2466/pms.1998.86.3.851.
11. Corlett PR, et al., *Trends Cogn Sci.* 2019. https://doi.org/10.1016/j.tics.2018.12.001.
12. Boksa P, On the neurobiology of hallucinations. *J Psychiatry Neurosci.* 2009;34(4):260–2.
13. Fisher CM, *Arch Neurol.* 1991. https://doi.org/10.1001/archneur.1991.00530220113031.
14. Peck T, et al., *Case Rep Med.* 2018. https://doi.org/10.1155/2018/5127917.
15. Desai S, et al., *Cureus.* 2021. https://doi.org/10.7759/cureus.17040.
16. Spanos NP, et al., *J Nerv Ment Dis.* 1979. https://doi.org/10.1097/00005053-197908000-00006.
17. El-Mallakh RS, et al., *Psych.* 2010. https://doi.org/10.1521/psyc.2010.73.1.34.
18. Kastaun S, et al., *J Cardiothorac Vasc Anesth.* 2016. https://doi.org/10.1053/j.jvca.2015.05.115.
19. Braun T, et al., *J Med Case Rep.* 2021. https://doi.org/10.1186/s13256-021-02902-6.
20. Penagaluri P, et al., *Crisis.* 2010. https://doi.org/10.1027/0227-5910/a000002.
21. Jacob A, et al., *BMJ.* 2004. https://doi.org/10.1136/bmj.328.7455.1552.
22. Kelson M, et al., *Psych R Case Rep.* 2022. http://doi.org/10.1016/j.psycr.2022.100036.
23. Berrios GE, *The History of Mental Symptoms: Descriptive Psychopathology Since the Nineteenth Century.* Cambridge, UK: Cambridge University Press; 1996: 35–70.
24. Aleman A, et al., *Hallucinations: The Science of Idiosyncratic Perception.* Washington DC: American Psychological Association; 2009: 25–46.
25. Bentall RP, *Madness Explained: Psychosis and Human Nature.* London: Penguin Books; 2003: 347–77.
26. Burde RM, et al., *Clinical Decisions in Neuro-Ophthalmology*, 3rd edn. St. Louis: Mosby; 2002: 114–35.
27. Norton JW, et al., *Semin Neurol.* 2000. https://doi.org/10.1055/s-2000-6837.
28. Spileers W, *Acta Ophthalmol.* 2009. https://doi.org/10.1111/j.1755-3768.2009.3421.x.
29. Tandon OP, et al., Visual evoked potentials in primary hypertension. *Indian J Physiol Pharmacol.* 1997;41(2):154–8.
30. Eisner A, et al., *J Opt Soc Am A Opt Image Sci Vis.* 2003. https://doi.org/10.1364/JOSAA.20.000569.
31. Walker CEL, et al., *J Neuroophthalmol.* 2025. https://doi.org/10.1097/WNO.0000000000002152.

32. Donat A, et al., *Rev Neurol (Paris)*. 2013. https://doi.org/10.1016/j.neurol.2012.05.015.
33. Thu WM, et al., *Eur J Case Rep Intern Med*. 2023. https://doi.org/10.12890/2023_003952.
34. Calvo-Maroto AM, et al., *Eye (Lond)*. 2014. https://doi.org/10.1038/eye.2014.176.
35. Applegate RA, et al., Entoptic evaluation of diabetic retinopathy. *Invest Ophthalmol Vis Sci*. 1997;38(5):783–91.
36. Levine AM, Visual hallucinations and cataracts. *Ophthalmic Surg*. 1980;11(2):95–8.
37. Harris KD, *Behav Brain Sci*. 2004. https://doi.org/10.1017/S0140525X04310186.
38. Feinberg I, *Schizophr Bull*. 2011. https://doi.org/10.1093/schbul/sbq115.

Chapter 4

ENTOPTIC PHENOMENA

Stefano Cena and Leonid Skorin, Jr.

Introduction

> "The intention is to stare into space to ease tired eyes but seeing more disturbs the tranquil spirit".[1]
>
> — **Ewald Hering**

Most of what we see reflects the external world. But not all of it. As you read the words on this page, light enters the eye through the cornea, passes through the aqueous humor, lens, and vitreous, and finally reaches the retina. There, specialized photoreceptors initiate a cascade of neural signals that the brain interprets as visual perception.

Some visual experiences originate from within the eye itself. These are known as *entoptic phenomena*—perceptions generated by the eye's own anatomy and physiology. Patients may describe them as shadows, floaters, flashes, or halos. Many are benign and transient. Others may be early signs of retinal or optic nerve pathology. Because these phenomena are internal, they are often highly subjective—varying from one patient to another and sometimes difficult to describe and, unfortunately, impossible to photograph.

In clinical practice, patients often struggle to describe these symptoms clearly. For eye care practitioners, recognizing the patterns of entoptic phenomena is essential to distinguish normal physiologic effects from visual disturbances that warrant urgent evaluation. Careful listening and thoughtful questioning are essential to interpreting these symptoms accurately and preventing potential vision loss. This chapter reviews the most common entoptic phenomena, their mechanisms, and their relevance to diagnosis and patient care.

Produced by the Eye's Own Structures

Halos Around Lights

i. Lens Fibers Act as a Diffraction Grating

Halos are luminous rings that patients notice when looking at bright light sources, usually when viewed from a distance, especially at night or in dim lighting. When the cause is the natural lens, halos tend to be due to light diffraction from the lenticular suture lines found in a healthy lens or early cataract formation. The lens fibers act as a radially arranged diffraction

DOI: 10.1201/9781003633365-4

grating, scattering incoming light into circular patterns.[2] The angular diameter of these physiologic halos ranges from 7°to 8° when measured to the outermost ring.[2] This figure is constant.[3] The color pattern is as follows: the short waved colors, blue and violet, are next to the stimulating light, with the long waves on the outside, with the orange and red forming the outermost rings (Figure 4.1).[2] Patients describe this effect as "glare" or "starbursts," particularly when driving at night or looking at streetlamps.

In early cataracts, halos can be the only visual complaint before noticeable visual acuity declines. These halos should be considered as pathologic halos and can occur from various pathological ocular conditions, including cataracts. Pathologic halos and physiologic halos are essentially identical regarding the color of the rainbow distribution, but physiologic halos are

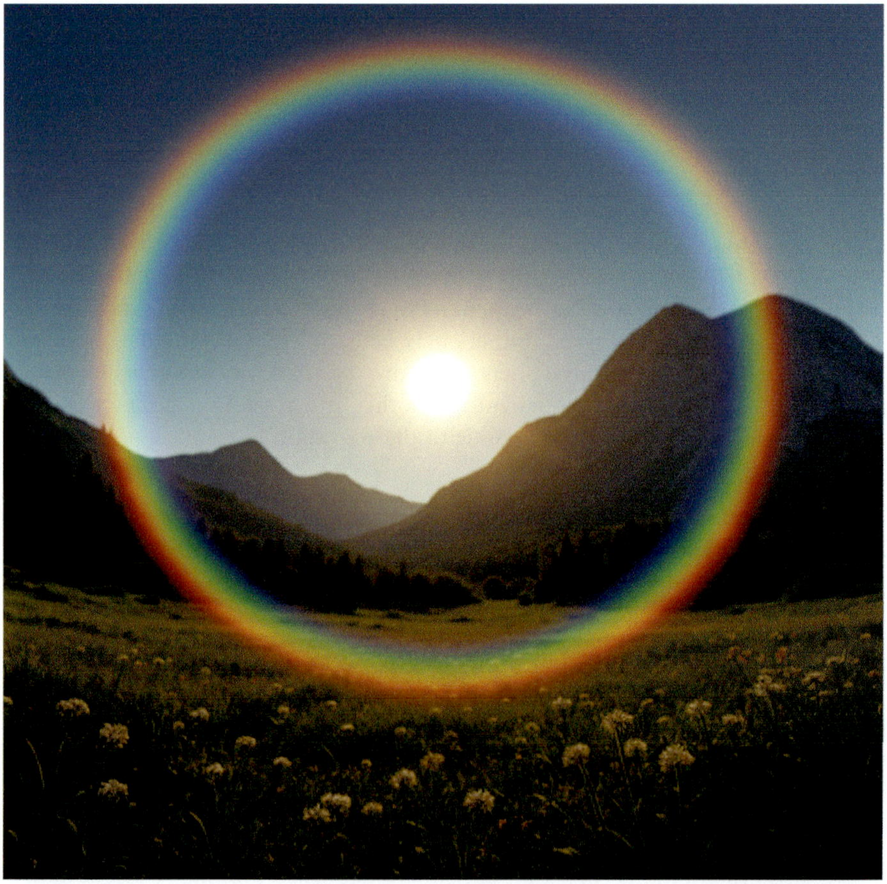

Figure 4.1 Halo Around Light Source: A visual representation of a photopic halo as perceived by individuals in low-light conditions or with corneal edema. The concentric glow surrounding the light source simulates diffraction and scattering of light on the corneal surface.

less bright as compared to pathologic halos.[2] Recognizing this symptom is important, especially when counseling patients about the progression of cataracts and the timing of surgical intervention.

ii. **Corneal Edema**

Corneal swelling can also cause halos by increasing light scatter. The cornea consists of five distinct layers: the epithelium, Bowman's layer, stroma, Descemet's membrane, and endothelium. The stroma comprises the bulk of the cornea and is made up of approximately 60 layers of collagen fibrils. Within each layer, fibrils are aligned in parallel, while the layers themselves are arranged perpendicularly to one another. This highly ordered, lattice-like structure is essential for corneal transparency, as the perpendicular arrangement minimizes light scatter. Flattened corneal fibroblasts reside between these layers and help maintain stromal structure and function.[4, 5]

When either the epithelium or endothelium is compromised (due to elevated intraocular pressure, endothelial dysfunction, or postoperative inflammation), fluid accumulates in the stroma, increasing hydration. This swelling disrupts the precise arrangement of collagen fibrils, leading to optical distortion, increased scatter, and loss of transparency. The result is visual phenomena such as diffraction and colored pathological halos from chromatic aberration.[5–7]

One simple way to picture this is the way light looks when reflected in a foggy bathroom mirror after a hot shower—it's diffused, blurred, and ringed by glare. Patients often notice these halos more in the morning or after rubbing their eyes.

Clinically, pathologic halos from corneal edema may be an early sign of acute angle-closure glaucoma, post-surgical corneal decompensation, contact lens overwear, or they may result from a corneal dystrophy such as Fuchs corneal endothelial dystrophy. The American Academy of Ophthalmology notes that in acute angle-closure glaucoma, corneal edema can present as halos around lights.[8] In some instances, after the underlying cause is addressed and the corneal edema resolves, visual acuity improves, and the pathologic halos disappear.[9, 10]

iii. **Dysphotopsias**

Dysphotopsias—unwanted optical phenomena—are a common source of postoperative dissatisfaction following cataract surgery. They are broadly categorized into negative and positive types, each with distinct characteristics and underlying mechanisms.

Negative Dysphotopsia

Negative dysphotopsia (ND) presents as a subjective, semilunar-shaped dark shadow, typically in the temporal peripheral visual field after posterior chamber intraocular lens (PCIOL) implantation. This phenomenon can be distressing for patients, even in cases with a well-centered PCIOL and uncomplicated surgical course.

The etiology of ND is multifactorial. While early theories implicated internal reflections, PCIOL edge design, and anterior capsule overlap, Holladay and Simpson's 2017 study[11] demonstrated that ray path geometry—how peripheral light rays are refracted or bypassed—plays a central role in ND development.

In a personal phone interview on March 26, 2025, Dr. Jack T. Holladay emphasized that while predicting ND with certainty is difficult, identifying patients at higher risk is possible[12]. He noted: "Just like we can look at risk factors that may lead to a heart attack but cannot predict exactly when an individual will have a heart attack, nobody can predict exactly when negative dysphotopsia will occur, but they can predict the individuals that are more likely to have negative dysphotopsia than others,"[12]

In their 2017 paper, Holladay and Simpson[11] ranked the following primary and secondary risk factors for ND in order of importance:

Primary Factors

- Smaller photopic pupil (approx. 2.5 mm)
- Larger positive angle kappa (angular difference between the visual and pupillary axes)
- Steeper posterior PCIOL surface
- Nasal anterior capsule overlying the anterior nasal PCIOL
- Higher PCIOL dioptric power if equi-biconvex or plano-convex surfaces
- PCIOL optic-haptic junction not horizontal (e.g., superonasal rotation by 30°)

Secondary Factors

- PCIOL edge design (truncated vs. rounded and edge thickness)
- Material used in PCIOL (e.g., acrylic lenses with higher index of refraction)
- PCIOLs containing negative aspheric surfaces

While a smaller photopic pupil was ranked highest in their model, Dr. Holladay emphasized that high PCIOL power and large angle kappa are often the most clinically actionable risk factors.[11, 12] These characteristics change how peripheral light enters the eye. Specifically, when temporal light rays bypass the optic entirely—passing through the space between the PCIOL and the iris—they may go unrefracted. Meanwhile, rays passing through the implanted lens are refracted. The result: a gap between refracted and unrefracted rays, producing a perceived temporal shadow. The higher the power or refractive index of the implanted lens, the greater the likelihood that this shadow will appear—and persist.[11, 12]

Large angle kappa is one of the most predictive anatomical features of ND.[11, 12] In patients with large angle kappa, peripheral rays enter at a more oblique angle and strike the nasal retina unevenly, increasing the risk of shadow perception.[11, 13–16]

These insights have clinical relevance. Holladay and colleagues demonstrated that acrylic PCIOLs—with their higher refractive index—enlarge the spatial zone behind the iris where shadows may form, raising the ND risk.[16] To mitigate this, surgeons may consider avoiding high-index lenses in patients with known risk factors, such as small photopic pupils or high angle kappa. Intraoperatively, careful attention to PCIOL centration, optic-haptic junction alignment, and nasal capsular overlap may reduce incidence. In some cases, reverse optic capture can prevent symptoms if performed at the time of surgery.[16]

According to the American Academy of Ophthalmology's *Cataract in the Adult Eye Preferred Practice Pattern*, the incidence of ND is approximately 15% on the first postoperative day, decreasing to 3% by one year without intervention.[17] Patients with intermittent symptoms are more likely to adapt over time, likely through neuroadaptation or capsular changes.

However, persistent ND does occur. Masket et al. reported that reverse optic capture and piggyback IOL implantation were effective in resolving persistent ND, with success rates of 21 out of 22 and 8 out of 11, respectively.[18] Makhotkina et al. found that approximately 1.5% of patients still experienced ND symptoms five years after surgery, although not all sought intervention.[19] When symptoms fail to improve within three to six months, surgical options—including reverse optic capture, silicone PCIOL exchange, or optic repositioning—may be considered.[20]

Positive & Multifocal Dysphotopsia

Positive dysphotopsias (PD) present differently, often as arcs, flashes, halos, or starbursts caused by oblique light interacting with PCIOL edge features.[20] The square-edge design is a primary contributor, causing internal reflection of light at the PCIOL periphery. Lenses with higher indices of refraction also increase PD likelihood, while a larger optic diameter may reduce its occurrence.[20] Multifocal dysphotopsias are distinct, frequently seen in diffractive implant platforms and often presenting as halos or concentric rings. Notably, patients may experience both PD and diffractive symptoms concurrently, complicating diagnosis and management. Cataract surgeons should identify all contributing components before proceeding with PCIOL exchange, as misattributing symptoms may result in inadequate surgical correction.[20] Exchanging to a silicone PCIOL—with a lower index of refraction—can reduce the risk of ND, as demonstrated in Holladay's study.[16] If appropriate, anteriorly shifting the implant's optic may further improve patient comfort.

Floaters

i. Muscae Volitantes

Muscae volitantes—Latin for "flitting flies" or *mouches volantes* (from the same phrase in French)—are small floating specks, wavy filaments or threads that drift across the visual field. They are particularly noticeable when patients look at bright, uniform backgrounds, such as a blue sky or white wall (Figure 4.2).[21] Patients will describe them as cobwebs, bugs, specks, spots, dots, string of beads, branching filaments, globules, or squiggles. These floaters seem to flit about like flies as the patient's line of

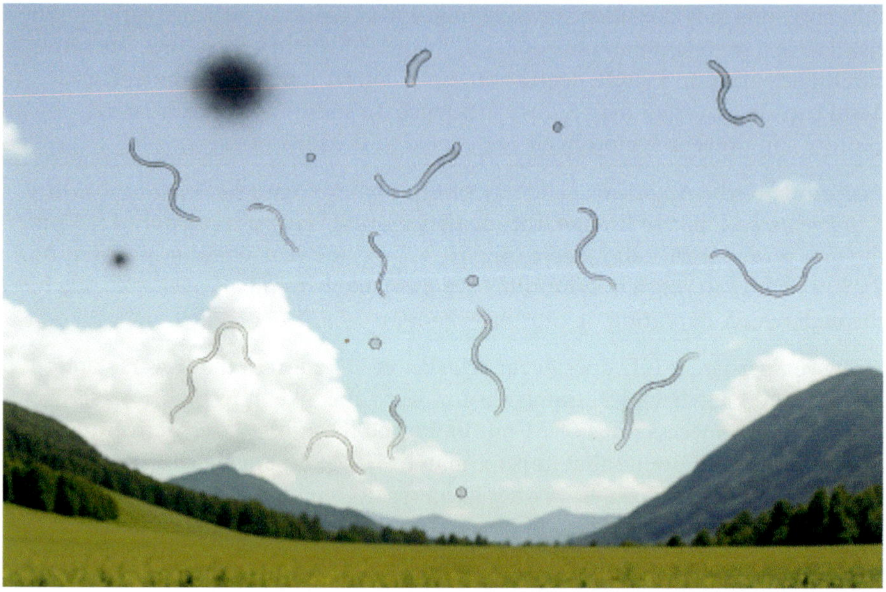

Figure 4.2 Muscae Volitantes (Floaters): A simulated depiction of vitreous floaters as seen against a bright background. The semi-transparent, threadlike, and globular shapes represent collagen fibrils casting shadows on the retina.

sight is oriented in various directions. It is difficult to actually visualize them since they tend to move away with attempted fixation.

In younger individuals, floaters typically result from cellular debris caused by small remnants of the embryonic hyaloid vascular system and later from age-related changes in the vitreous humor. Over time, the vitreous undergoes liquefaction and syneresis (contraction of the vitreous gel with separation of some of its fluid), leading to the aggregation of collagen fibrils and hyalocytes. These suspended clumps scatter light and cast moving shadows on the retina, producing the illusion of mobile visual artifacts.[21,22] Since the vitreous never circulates or gets replenished, these floaters persist forever. With time, these floaters may break down into smaller, less noticeable segments to which many patients can more readily neuroadapt.

Although floaters are often benign, a sudden onset of floaters, especially when accompanied by photopsia (flashing lights), may indicate a posterior vitreous detachment (PVD) or a retinal break-tear (see Illustrative Case at the end of the chapter).[23] The patient with an acute retinal tear will still have a complete visual field.[24] Approximately 8% to 10% of all patients with an acute symptomatic PVD have a retinal break.[25] The presence of pigmented cells in the anterior vitreous with an acute PVD indicates a high probability of a coexisting retinal break.[25] In acute cases, the fundus must be thoroughly examined with pharmacological dilation of the pupil to assess the retina and rule out retinal breaks, which may progress to retinal detachment if untreated.[26]

In those patients without any retinal involvement, reassurance about their floaters is sufficient. As mentioned previously, floaters tend to become less noticeable over time due to both neuroadaptation and gradual disintegration with movement away from the visual axis.[27] However, in selective cases where floaters impair visual function or quality of life, treatment should be considered.

Two primary treatment modalities exist:

- Laser vitreolysis, which uses a Nd:YAG laser to disrupt and vaporize floaters. Results are variable, and potential risks include retinal damage or increased floaters.[28]
- Pars plana vitrectomy, a surgical removal of the vitreous, is more definitive but carries higher risks, including retinal detachment, cataract formation, and endophthalmitis.[29]

Both procedures should be reserved for carefully selected patients after conservative management has failed, and symptoms remain functionally limiting.

ii. Scheerer's Phenomenon

Scheerer's phenomenon, also known as flying spots, flying corpuscles, or blue-field entoptic phenomena, represents the visualization of white blood cells (leukocytes) moving through the retinal capillaries near the fovea. Since the fovea is an avascular zone, the movement of these leukocytes cannot be seen exactly at the point the patient fixates.[30] The specific retinal vessel etiology has been identified as the capillary loop of the inner nuclear/outer plexiform layers of the retina.[31] It is best seen when a patient gazes at a bright blue sky and perceives tiny, bright whitish spots or "tadpoles" darting quickly in short, curved paths and leaving a tail, like a comet. These spots were initially thought to be red blood cells (thus the name flying corpuscles).[30] Since blue light is absorbed by hemoglobin, which is found in red blood cells, it is now thought that these spots represent the passage of leukocytes through capillaries since they allow blue light to pass through them.[32, 33] In addition, the spots seen in any one field selected for observation are not sufficiently numerous to be red blood cells.[30] This is a normal physiologic process that is rarely noticed unless deliberately observed.[32] Applying pressure to the globe makes them easier to see, and they can be observed to move in a pulsatile fashion that accelerates with an increased heart rate.[31]

This entoptic effect is often cited in ophthalmic physiology, is non-pathologic and can be used clinically as evidence of a normally functioning macula. Using a specialty instrument known as the blue-field entoptoscope, macular function in cataract patients can be assessed. Studies have shown that this instrument can predict good macular function in patients with dense cataracts, but it is even more accurate in predicting poor macular function.[34] The reliability of the test decreases with increased cataract opacity. The test is also subjective, and, therefore, results depend on the patient's understanding of what they are looking for and being able to communicate this information to the cataract surgeon. The test is of little use with significant vitreous opacity.[35]

iii. Shafer's Sign (Tobacco Dust)

Shafer's sign, also known as tobacco dust, refers to the presence of brown-pigmented cells floating in the anterior vitreous. These are typically pigment granules originating from the retinal pigment epithelium and are visible on slit-lamp biomicroscopy. Their presence is highly suggestive of a retinal break or tear and warrants an urgent peripheral retinal examination through a pharmacologically dilated pupil. Unlike benign floaters, Shafer's sign carries significant clinical diagnostic weight and is a red flag in patients presenting with new-onset floaters or flashes.

Phosphenes—Flashes of Light

i. Retinal Stimulation

Phosphenes are the perception of light without an actual light source. This makes phosphenes (seeing light from a non-light stimulus) different from all the other entoptic phenomena. They may result from mechanical or electrical stimulation of the retina or visual cortex. If the phosphenes are a result of mechanical stimulation (rubbing your closed eyes), this occurs from an increase in vitreous pressure on and deformation of the retina. Vitreoretinal traction—such as during PVD—can also mechanically stimulate photoreceptors, producing the illusion of light flashes. These are often located in the periphery and are of brief duration. This is an important symptom, especially if accompanied by new-onset floaters, in the early detection of retinal tears or detachment, and should be investigated thoroughly.

ii. Prolonged Accommodation

Extended screen use, prolonged close-up tasks, or sustained ciliary muscle contraction can occasionally cause visual aftereffects, such as brief flashes or shimmering. The mechanism is unclear but may involve changes in intraocular pressure or local retinal metabolism. These are typically self-limited and resolve with rest.

iii. Quick Eye Movement

Rapid saccadic movements can occasionally stretch and deform the vitreous, momentarily stimulating the retina and causing the nerve fibers in the region to fire, producing a brief phosphene. This is more noticeable in older patients with vitreous syneresis, where the vitreous becomes less viscous. It is known as a flick phosphene and is best observed by the fully dark-adapted eye.[36] Patients often see these phosphenes upon awakening and describe them as a bright streak that is sheaf-like in shape.[37]

iv. Digitally Pressing the Eye

Applying pressure to a closed eyelid can produce diffuse or focal phosphene sensations, often perceived as shimmering lights or bursts of color (Figure 4.3). This classic demonstration of retinal excitability reinforces the principle that photoreceptors—and possibly downstream retinal neurons—can be activated by non-photic mechanical stimuli. Everyone has experienced this at some point, whether from rubbing tired eyes or accidental pressure on

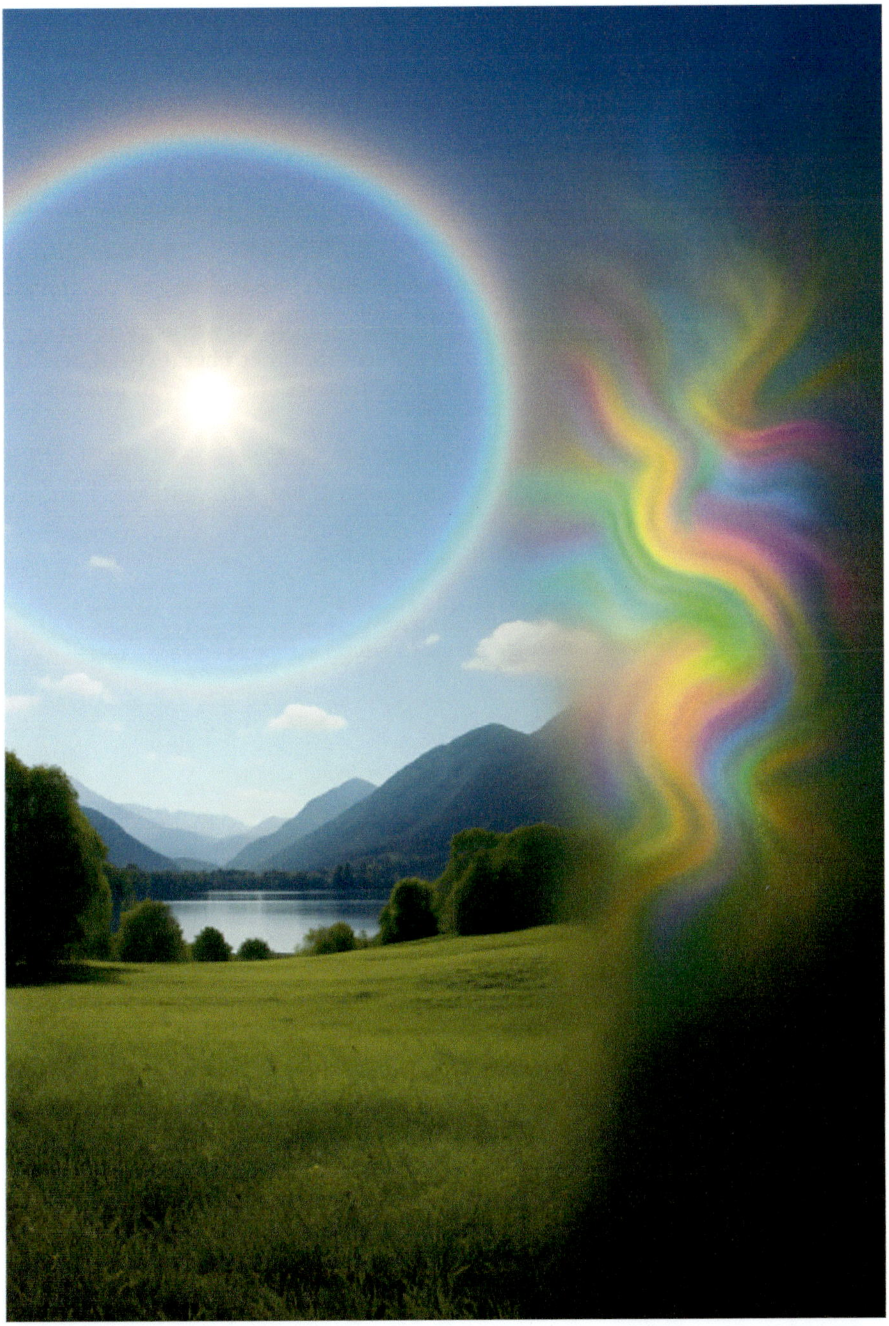

Figure 4.3 Phosphenes Induced by Digital Pressure on Right Lateral Canthus: Simulation of phosphene phenomenon produced by pressing on a closed eyelid. The colorful arcs and bursts in the peripheral visual field represent mechanically induced stimulation of the retina, independent of light.

the globe. While benign, this phenomenon highlights the retina's sensitivity and the brain's tendency to interpret any retinal stimulation—regardless of source—as visual information. Infants with poor vision are thought to rub their eyes in order to trigger phosphenes and stimulate the optic nerve.

Clinically, this is important during visual acuity or confrontation visual field testing—care should be taken to avoid inadvertent pressure on the globe. Cupping the hand properly over the eye helps prevent mechanically induced phosphenes from confounding the patient's responses.

v. Moore's Lightning Streaks

First described by R. F. Moore in 1935, these unformed vertical streaks usually, but not exclusively appear in the temporal peripheral visual field of elderly patients (Figure 4.4).[38] They occur more commonly in females

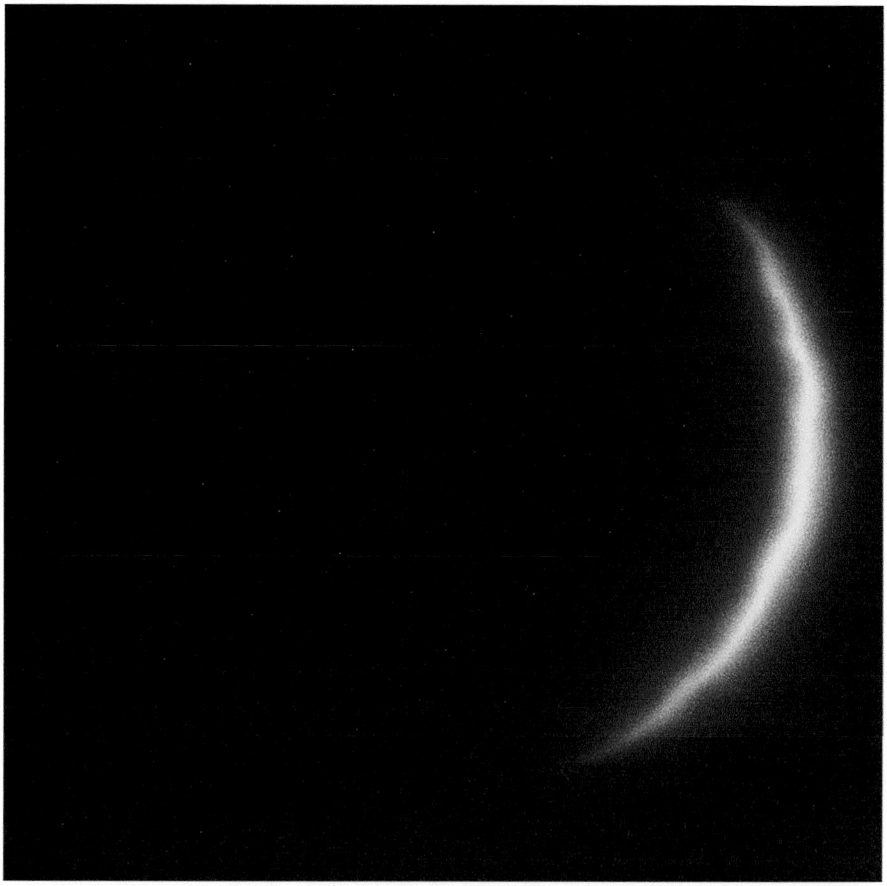

Figure 4.4 Moore's Lightning Streaks: A simulation of peripheral photopsia caused by vitreoretinal traction, commonly observed in posterior vitreous detachment. The bright, jagged streaks extending vertically across the peripheral temporal visual field illustrate the classic "lightning streak" pattern described by Moore.

than males and are associated with a few vitreous opacities.[37] They are often noticed in low light or during rapid eye movement and are attributed to vitreoretinal traction from vitreous shrinkage in the peripheral retina.[39] Traction on the temporal retina near the ora serrata may not be noted subjectively by the patient since the periphery of the temporal retina is blind, while similar traction on the seeing peripheral nasal retina may be observed as a phosphene referred to the temporal visual field.[39] Although often benign, their presence warrants evaluation for retinal pathology such as retinal detachment.[37, 40]

Light-Induced Visual Disturbances

i. Purkinje Tree

The retinal blood vessels lie in front of the photoreceptors and cast a shadow upon them because of their near proximity. And yet, under normal conditions of illumination, patients do not see these vessels even though they are there all the time. This is because the visual cortex can separate self from non-self—a form of neuroadaptation to these permanent, stationary blood vessels branching patterns. It takes a significantly brighter amount of, and direction change in, illumination to stimulate the underlying photoreceptors, thus visualizing the shadows cast by the retinal vasculature onto the retina. In addition, since stable images on the retina quickly fade (Troxler phenomenon), the branching retinal arterioles and venules are best seen if a light source constantly moves over a large angle. The best light sources to use in clinic are the slit-lamp biomicroscope and the binocular indirect ophthalmoscope. The illumination from these instruments is brighter than most standard light sources that typically enter the eye. Also, the light sources of both instruments can be constantly kept in motion, stimulating the different underlying photoreceptors from different angles and preventing their neuroadaptation. As the light source is moved, the tree branch-like image that is seen in the visual field will move correspondingly.[41] The interlacing branches of the retinal vessels resemble a black tree branch-like lacework against a red background.[42]

ii. Exposure to Intense Modern LED Headlights

With the widespread adoption of light-emitting diode (LED) and high-intensity discharge (HID) headlights in newer vehicles, patients have increasingly reported symptoms of glare, transient halos, and afterimages when driving at night. These lights emit a higher proportion of blue-spectrum light, which scatters more readily in the eye and can overwhelm the dark-adapted retina.[43]

Although not strictly entoptic—since they originate from external sources—these effects interact with the eye's internal optics and can mimic or exacerbate entoptic symptoms such as halos and afterimages. Disabling glare, photostress, and delayed recovery times are often more pronounced in older patients, those with early natural lens changes, or following refractive surgery.[43]

While headlight brightness and beam alignment are regulated by standards such as FMVSS 108 in the United States and Economic Commission of Europe regulations in Europe, the spectral composition of automotive lighting—particularly the proportion of short-wavelength blue light—remains largely unregulated. This matters because blue light scatters more (Rayleigh scatter), causes greater glare, and can increase retinal photostress, especially under scotopic (dark-adapted) conditions.[43] Although blue light-induced phototoxicity remains debated, its potential to impair visual function during night driving is clinically relevant.[44]

Currently, there are no specific limits on blue light emission from vehicle headlights. Given the growing number of patient complaints, further investigation and regulatory attention may be warranted.[43]

Conclusion

Entoptic phenomena represent a spectrum of visual experiences arising from the eye's internal structures and physiology. From benign floaters and phosphenes to diagnostically significant signs like Shafer's sign or symptoms like negative dysphotopsia, recognizing these effects helps clinicians distinguish normal from pathological states and respond appropriately.

Clinicians are often the first to validate visual experiences that patients struggle to articulate. A clear understanding of these subtle phenomena allows eye care practitioners not only to reassure patients but also to detect early signs of potentially serious conditions.

As surgical techniques, lighting environments, and imaging technologies evolve, so does our ability to detect and contextualize entoptic disturbances. Tools like ray-tracing simulations and artificial intelligence-assisted diagnostics are beginning to reveal optical subtleties that can guide both diagnosis and surgical planning.[18, 45] Continued research in these areas may further personalize and refine patient care.

Illustrative Case

A 67-year-old male was seen at the eye clinic after he experienced an episode of new-onset floaters and flashes earlier that same day. He was sitting quietly while watching a television show when suddenly in his right eye he noticed a flash of light and a dark globule in his central vision. This dark globule, which appeared opaque, seemed to flow slowly "like dirty oil or sludge" in an upward direction, "like one would see in a lava lamp". It persisted for a couple of minutes, dissipated and left multiple smaller floaters in its wake. There was also a larger, more distinct ring-like floater which readily moved with eye excursions. He denied any eye pain during this visual episode. The patient denied any recent eye or head trauma. He was not a diabetic and was otherwise healthy except for having high cholesterol which was readily controlled with daily anti-cholesterol medication.

On visual evaluation, the patient could read at distance 20/25 right eye and 20/20 left eye through his most recent compound myopic astigmatic spectacle correction. He mentioned that his vision would blur intermittently as he was trying to read the Snellen chart with his right eye whenever the swath of floaters would get into his visual axis. His pupils, ocular motility, confrontation visual fields and intraocular pressures were all normal. Slit-lamp biomicroscopy was unremarkable and there was no tobacco dust (Shafer's sign) in the anterior vitreous. A thorough pharmacological dilated fundus examination indicated no retinal holes, tears, breaks, hemorrhages or detachment. The vitreous cavity showed a complete Weiss ring (ring-like floater) and multiple smaller floaters appearing to be in a sheet of detached vitreous, none of which was a hemorrhage. A Weiss ring is peripapillary glial tissue which can be visualized by both the clinician (with ophthalmoscopy) and the patient if it is pulled off the optic disc rim during a PVD.[46]

The patient was reassured that he did not have a retinal detachment. He was told that he had experienced a PVD, and although it was generally benign in nature, there likely would be persistence of his floaters. He was counseled to minimize his physical activity over the next several weeks. He was told to return immediately if he noted any persistent flashes of light, worsening in his vision, occurrence of any curtain or scotoma in his field of vision, or any new additional onset of floaters or change in their appearance. It is recommended to see these patients in four to six weeks and periodically thereafter.[45]

At his six-week follow-up visit, subjectively, the patient noted a slight decrease in his floaters and no new flashes of light or curtain, or scotoma in his field of vision. He felt his vision was relatively normal except when the Weiss ring entered the center of his line of sight. Objectively, the patient could read 20/20 with his right eye through his spectacles whenever the Weiss ring was not in his visual axis. The slit-lamp examination indicated no evidence of tobacco dust (Shafer's sign). A dilated fundus examination was negative for any untoward retinal pathology such as detachment. The patient was again counseled, as before, and scheduled for an annual eye examination.

REFERENCES

1. Attributed to Ewald Hering, paraphrased from *Outlines of a Theory of the Light Sense. Hering E, Outlines of a Theory of the Light Sense.* Trans. Hurvich LM, Jameson D. Cambridge, MA: Harvard University Press, 1964.
2. Miller KM, et al., *Ophthalmology.* 2022. https://doi.org/10.1016/j.ophtha.2021.10.006.
3. van den Berg TJTP, *Ophthal Physiol Opt.* https://doi.org/10.1111/opo.12426.
4. Meek KM, et al., *Eye.* 2025. https://doi.org/10.1038/s41433-024-02969-7.
5. Meek KM, et al., *Biophys J.* 2003. https://doi.org/10.1016/S0006-3495(03)74646-3.

6. Briceno-Lopez C, et al., *J Clin Med.* 2023. https://doi.org/10.3390/jcm12216751.
7. He F, et al., *Physiol Res.* 2019. https://doi.org/10.33549/physiolres.934011.
8. Gedde SJ, et al., *Ophthalmology.* 2021. https://doi.org/10.1016/j.ophtha.2020.10.021.
9. Wacker K, et al., *Cornea.* 2018. https://doi.org/10.1097/ICO.0000000000001465.
10. Loreck N, et al., *Am J Ophthalmol.* 2020. https://doi.org/10.1016/j.ajo.2020.01.011.
11. Holladay JT, et al., Negative dysphotopsia: Causes and rationale for prevention and treatment. *J Cataract Refract Surg.* 2017;43(2):263–75.
12. Holladay JT, Personal phone interview. March 26, 2025.
13. Masket S, et al., Pseudophakic negative dysphotopsia: Surgical management and new theory of etiology. *J Cataract Refract Surg.* 2011;37(7):1199–205.
14. Osher RH, Negative dysphotopsia: Long-term study and possible explanation for transient symptoms. *J Cataract Refract Surg.* 2008;34(10):1699–707.
15. Olson RJ, Angle kappa and its importance in intraocular lens centration. *J Cataract Refract Surg.* 2001;27(3):419.
16. Holladay JT, Comment on pseudophakic negative dysphotopsia: Surgical management and new theory of etiology. *J Cataract Refract Surg.* 2013;39(3):400.
17. Miller KM, et al., *Ophthalmology.* 2022. https://doi.org/10.1016/j.ophtha.2021.10.006.
18. Masket S, et al., *J Cataract Refract Surg.* 2018. https://doi.org/10.1016/j.jcrs.2017.10.038.
19. Makhotkina NY, et al., *Acta Ophthalmol.* 2018. https://doi.org/10.1111/aos.13508.
20. Hunter L, *Investigating IOL complaints. Rev Ophthalmol.* 2025;4:43–8. Available from: https://www.reviewofophthalmology.com/article/investigating-iol-complaints.
21. Harmer SW, et al., *Bioelectromagnetics.* 2022. https://doi.org/10.1002/bem.22386.
22. Sebag J, *Am J Ophthalmol.* 2011. https://doi.org/10.1016/j.ajo.2011.02.015.
23. Byer NE, Clinical study of posterior vitreous detachment with early management of retinal breaks. *Trans Am Ophthalmol Soc.* 1994;92:125–44.
24. Kreissig I, *A Practical Guide to Minimal Surgery for Retinal Detachment.* Vol. 1. Stuttgart: Thieme; 2000: 1–6.
25. Ehlers JP, Shah CP, *eds, The Wills Eye Manual*, 5th edn. Philadelphia: Wolters Kluwer; 2008: 274–279.
26. Royal Australian College of General Practitioners, Flashes and floaters. *Aust Fam Physician.* 2014;43(4):205–7.
27. Webb BF, et al., Patient perceptions of eye floaters. *Am J Ophthalmol.* 2013;155(6):1034–8.

28. Singh IP, et al., Nd:YAG laser vitreolysis for symptomatic vitreous floaters: safety, efficacy, and patient satisfaction. *Int Ophthalmol.* 2020;40(4):873–9.
29. Delaney YM, et al., Vitrectomy for floaters: prospective efficacy analyses and retrospective safety profile. *Br J Ophthalmol.* 2002;86(6):744–6.
30. Loebl M, et al., *Ophthalmology.* 1978. https://doi.org/10.1016/s0161-6420(78)35599-8.
31. Fuchsjäger-Mayrl G, et al., Effects of granulocyte colony stimulating factor on retinal leukocyte and erythrocyte flux in the human retina. *Invest Ophthalmol Vis Sci.* 2002;43(5):1520–4.
32. Kolodjaschna J, et al., *Am J Physiol.* 2004. https://doi.org/10.1152/ajpheart.01240.2003.
33. Zetlan SR, et al., Retinal capillary hemodynamics, visual-evoked potentials, and pressure tolerance in normal human eyes. *Invest Ophthalmol Vis Sci.* 1992;33(6):1857–63.
34. Riva CE, et al., Autoregulation of blood flow in the capillaries of the human macula. *Invest Ophthalmol Vis Sci.* 1977;16(6):568–71.
35. Tanaka T, et al., *Ophthalmology.* 1991. https://doi.org/10.1016/s0161-6420(91)32043-8.
36. Marshall C, Entoptic phenomena associated with the retina. *Br J Ophthalmol.* 1935;19:177–201.
37. Nebel BR, The phosphene of quick eye motion. *Arch Ophthalmol.* 1957;58:235–43.
38. Kassoff A, Flashes, floaters, and posterior vitreous detachment. Focal Points: Clinical Modules for Ophthalmologists. *Am. Acad. Ophthalmol.* 2004;22:1–14.
39. Verhoeff FH, "Are Moore's lightning streaks of serious portent? *Am J Ophthalmol.* 1956;41(5):837–40.
40. Berens C, et al., Moore's lightning streaks: A discussion of their innocuousness. *Trans Am Ophthalmol Soc.* 1954;52:35–63.
41. Luckiesh M, *Visual Illusions: Their Causes, Characteristics & Applications.* New York: Dover Publications; 1965: 27.
42. Adams DL, et al., *J Neurosci.* 2003. https://doi.org/10.1523/JNEUROSCI.23-14-05984.2003.
43. Behar-Cohen F, et al., *Prog Retin Eye Res.* 2011. https://doi.org/10.1016/j.preteyeres.2011.04.002.
44. O'Hagan JB, et al., *Eye.* 2016;30(2):230–3. https://doi.org/10.1038/eye.2015.261.
45. Grulkowski I, et al., *Biomed Opt Express.* 2021.
46. Jaffe NS, et al., *Cataract Surgery and its Complications*, 5th edn. Saint Louis: C.V. Mosby; 1990: 3–20.

Chapter 5

ILLUSIONS

Leonid Skorin, Jr. and Zachary Dwyer

Introduction

"Try to see it my way.[1]"

—The Beatles

An illusion can be simply defined as the misperception of a viewed object or scene. For example, a patient may interpret a snake hanging from a tree when in reality it was just a rope. Therefore, this patient is actually experiencing a "false impression" of the object or scene being viewed. Illusions are commonly contrasted against hallucinations, the topic of Chapter 7. Hallucinations are the perception of something that is not physically present, such as seeing a person walking by the window when no one is actually there. One easy way to differentiate between the two is that if the patient closes their eyes and the image disappears, the false perception is an illusion. Both illusions and hallucinations can be due to dysfunction of the visual pathway, including the retina, optic nerve, and occipital lobe. However, illusions can also be due to other pathologies such as cataracts, vitreous hemorrhage, or medication side effects.[2]

When working up a patient with altered visual perceptions, the first step should be to distinguish whether the patient is perceiving a hallucination or an illusion. Once the visual perception has been established as an illusion, the next best step is defining what type of illusion it is. This should help narrow the differential and point to the correct etiology. The rest of this chapter will be focused on describing the different illusions and helping establish the etiology and formulate subsequent management.

Not all visual illusions are due to ocular or intracranial disease. Most are visual aberrations due to natural light wave functioning, misinterpretation because of a difficult visual environment (inadequate illumination of the viewed object or event), our own visual system's physiological structural shortcomings (anatomical shape and structure of the natural lens), and, finally, our own inherent capacity to misconstrue perfectly adequate sensory signs. Before further discussing the clinically relevant visual illusions, it would be of interest to illustrate some common natural and artificially produced nonpathological visual illusions. The natural function of light rays takes into account that as light travels through different matter, light slows down.[3] How much the light slows down in a given medium is represented by that medium's index of refraction.[3] Therefore, a light

DOI: 10.1201/9781003633365-5

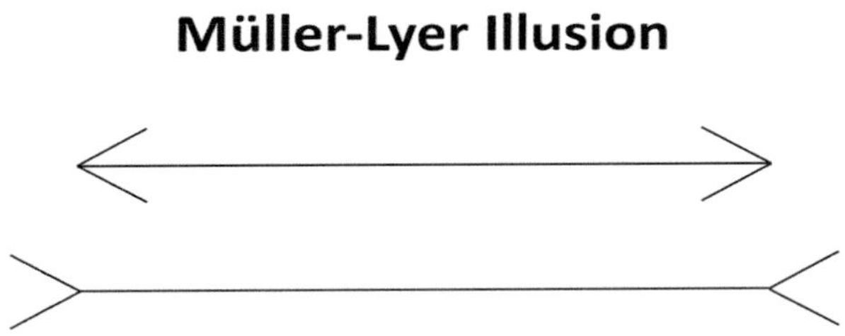

Figure 5.1 Müller-Lyer Illusion where the two horizontal lines are the same length, but the direction of the arrows creates an illusion of different-sized horizontal lines. The line with the inward-pointing arrowheads appears to be longer than the line with the outward-pointing arrowheads.

ray which is travelling in a straight line through air will be bent at the surface of a second transparent medium, such as water, as it enters the water. This is why a straw in a glass of water appears to be bent or broken. Another natural illusion is the moon illusion where the size of the moon appears to be considerably larger on the horizon than it does at higher elevations toward the zenith of the sky.[4] And yet, photographs of the horizon moon and zenith moon taken with the same camera settings yield images which are the same size.[4] Multiple theories have been proposed for this phenomenon. One theory revolves around various cues placing the horizon moon at a greater distance than the elevated moon.[5] A newer theory points towards accommodation causing the zenith moon to appear smaller.[5] The best known artificial visual illusion is the Müller-Lyer (Figure 5.1).[6] This artificially produced illusion consists of two parallel lines of equal length: one of these ends in inward-pointing arrowheads, the other in outward-pointing arrowheads. The visual illusion occurs when the individual viewing these two lines sees the line with the inward-pointing arrowheads as appearing to be longer than the line with the outward-pointing arrowheads. False line length interpretation occurs as a result of the misleading cues given by the influence of angles and the direction of the different arrowheads.[7]

Multiple Images

If a patient is complaining of seeing two of the same images, they have diplopia; if they see more than two of the same images, this is polyopia. In cases of diplopia, the clinician must differentiate whether the patient has monocular or binocular diplopia. The simplest first test to do is to ask the patient to close one eye at a time. In binocular diplopia cases, the second image will disappear when the patient closes either eye. This usually indicates the disruption of the ocular motor system, involving the extraocular muscles, nerves or supranuclear pathways. In monocular diplopia, the double vision originates solely from one eye so when the patient closes the affected eye, the double vision disappears but persists when the unaffected eye is closed.[8] To further refine the etiology of the monocular diplopia, the pinhole test should be performed. While using a pinhole occluder, the patient positions it in front of the affected eye. If the

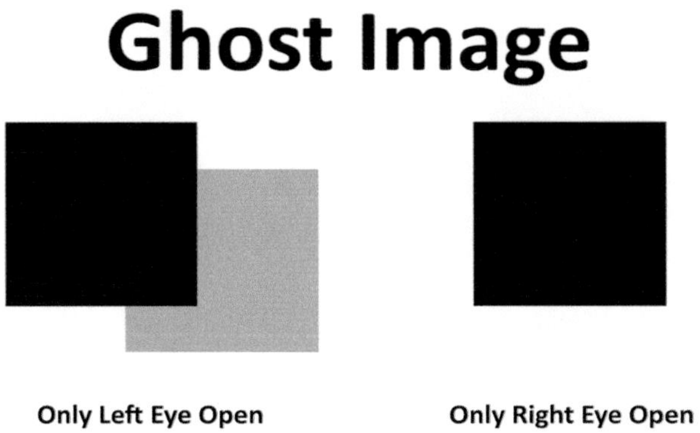

Figure 5.2 Monocular diplopia observed in the left eye with ghost image seen adjacent to the true image.

image duplication disappears then the underlying cause is likely an ocular media aberration or uncorrected refractive error. The pinhole functions by allowing only the paraxial central light rays to enter through the cornea perpendicular to the corneal surface, thus eliminating any peripheral distortions or reflections.[9] Many of these diplopic images may more appropriately be called "ghost images" where the second false image is a poorly focused spectral image adjacent to the clearer true image.[8, 10] The true image of the single object falls on the fovea and extra-foveal retina simultaneously, creating the sharper and "ghost image" respectively (Figure 5.2).[11]

There are many potential etiologies which can cause monocular diplopia. They can result from refractive errors such as irregular astigmatism and myopia. One possible cause of an irregular astigmatism is a long-standing chalazion that hardens and impinges on the corneal surface distorting the corneal refractive structure. Physiologic diplopia can occur in myopic patients when they look through their glasses in peripheral directions.[12] Spectacle lenses that correct for myopia are known as minus power lenses; they are concave-shaped with the edge thickness of the ophthalmic lens being greater than its center thickness.[13] An ophthalmic lens is composed of a series of many prisms; in a minus lens, these prisms are specifically aligned apex to apex.[14] Prisms bend (refract) visible light toward their base which in the minus lens is toward the periphery of the ophthalmic lens.[14] Therefore, a myopes glasses will refract visible light rays to the periphery and objects visible outside the glasses may appear twice through the margin of the spectacle ophthalmic lens.[12] Other device-induced monocular diplopia can result from a decentered contact lens, displaced intraocular lens implant, improperly positioned bifocal segment line or double reflection within a glasses ophthalmic lens. Medical issues such as blepharitis eyelid infection, excessive tearing, and ocular surface changes which can cause tear film disruption from dry eye syndrome may cause monocular diplopia.[8] Corneal structural diseases such as keratoconus which may induce irregular astigmatism and Fuchs' corneal endothelial dystrophy which can cause significant corneal edema are common corneal pathologies that cause monocular diplopia. Other intraocular causes include abnormalities of the iris such as polycoria, traumatic iridodialysis, and large laser-induced iridotomies (to correct narrow occludable angles and prevent angle-closure glaucoma), multi-refractile cataracts which may contain vacuoles and clefts causing additional symptoms of decreased visual acuity, haze and glare, and retinal pathology such as cystoid macular edema, epiretinal membrane (ERM), choroidal neovascular membrane seen in exudative macular degeneration and idiopathic central serous retinopathy, all of which physically distort or displace the fovea and cause metamorphopsia (see Chapter 7).[8, 15] A binocular diplopia known as dragged fovea diplopia syndrome may also potentially develop due to wrinkling of the macula (macular pucker) or following the surgical intervention to correct the ERM with vitrectomy and membrane peel.[16] Rarer causes include the development of anomalous retinal correspondence from strabismus surgery and neurological diseases with unilateral disc papilledema such as in idiopathic intracranial hypertension (IIH).[11] In the case of the unilateral disc edema from IIH, the underlying pathology is assumed to be caused by transudation of the cerebral spinal fluid through the nerve fibers into the macula causing a change in the dioptric media.[11] Papilledema, by definition, is bilateral disc edema; in unusual situations, however, it can occur unilaterally in about 10% of patients with IIH.[11, 17]

Monocular diplopia is not as common as binocular diplopia and represents between 11.5% and 25% of all cases of diplopia.[18, 19] It should be mentioned that if the pinhole test does not eliminate the image duplication and there is no provable posterior visual pathway disease, the etiology may actually be a functional disorder (psychogenic, pretend non-organic diplopia).[10, 12] All true diplopic images tilt when the patient tilts their head. As an example, if the diplopic images present horizontally when the patient is maintaining an upright head position, then the images will be nearly vertical in a 90° ear down, parallel to the floor position.[12] If the orientation of the diplopic images never changes even as the patient positions their head at various angles then a functional or non-organic origin should be suspected.[12] Another unusual presentation can occur when a patient exhibits bilateral monocular diplopia resulting from a primary or secondary visual cortex disorder.[20] This has been described in patients who see more than two images, as in cerebral polyopia (see Chapter 6).[20] Unlike unilateral monocular diplopia due to ocular media aberrations, cerebral diplopia is present and identical in both eyes, usually accompanied by visual field defects or other cerebral visual disorders and is not eliminated by pinhole.[21] Bilateral monocular diplopia has been described in patients with perseveration of vision (palinopsia) where multiple images appear in the visual scene soon after the gaze has been turned away from an object or after it has been removed from view (see Chapter 6).[20] Palinopsia is also associated with hemifield defects.[21]

Treatment includes correcting any existing refractive error with glasses, contact lenses, or refractive surgery.[15] Artificial tear drop supplements, gels, or punctal occlusion can be used for ocular surface disease as seen in dry eye syndrome. If irregular astigmatism arises from the corneal surface, then rigid gas permeable or scleral contact lenses may help. If refractive correction is not helpful, a topical miotic agent such as pilocarpine may attenuate the diplopia.[10] Corneal distortion can be documented and graded with manual keratometry or corneal topography. Corneal cross-linking can be performed to slow or halt the progression of keratoconus.[22] Cataracts can be corrected with phacoemulsification and intraocular lens implant placement. Sometimes just increasing the amount of ambient light may minimize the "ghost image" to a point where the patient can learn to ignore it.

Altered Size or Shape

When an individual needs no corrective glasses or contact lenses to see well, they are considered to have emmetropia and the image of a distant object that they are viewing is brought to focus equally on the fovea of both eyes. If an individual has a refractive error such as myopia, hyperopia, or astigmatism they have ametropia and a distant viewed object no longer focuses equally on their foveas. It is the existence of these refractive errors and their correction, especially with spectacles, that may lead to illusions of altered size, shape or tilt. These illusions may occur in patients who have a difference in ophthalmic lens dioptric power between the two eyes.[23] This difference in refractive errors between the two eyes is known as anisometropia and may become clinically significant in the amount of 1.00 diopter or more.[24] The correction with spectacle lenses of the anisometropia may lead to headache, asthenopia, dizziness, photophobia, reading difficulties, visual distortion and altered size, shape, and tilt illusions.[23, 25] These clinical problems may develop when a patient with anisometropia has received their first spectacle correction, or if there is a significant refractive change which warrants an ophthalmic lens change in their habitual glasses. The resulting foveal images between the two eyes develop an inequality in the ocular images involving their size, shape, tilt or even brightness.[25] This inequality of ocular images is known as aniseikonia and patients will complain that they see images of different sizes and shapes between their two eyes.[23, 25–27] As discussed in the previous section on Multiple Images, all ophthalmic lenses are composed of a series of many prisms. Minus lenses that are used to correct myopia are composed of prisms that are aligned apex to apex and cause image minification.[14] Plus lenses that are used to correct hyperopia are composed of prisms that are aligned base to base and cause image magnification.[14] A prism will bend visible light toward its base.[13] All these ophthalmic lenses will bend (refract), visible light to varying degrees resulting in potential image blur seen by the patient.[13] In addition to the potential occurrence of image size and shape differences, anisometropia can cause illusions because of this prismatic effect inherent in the construction of the ophthalmic lenses themselves.[23, 25] This is known as anisophoria, which is a heterophoria that varies with gaze from one direction to another.[23, 25–27] In clinical practice, the induced prism through spectacle lenses, and the resultant anisophoria in different directions of gaze, is nearly always more of a problem than image size differences.[23]

There are many ways to avoid or minimize anisometropia, aniseikonia, and anisophoria and, therefore, eliminate (or at least minimize) the resultant visual illusions. If a patient is having difficulty adjusting to the new anisometropic-correcting spectacle refraction, partial correction with temporary spectacles, slip-on lenses or Fresnel stick-on lenses can be tried with a gradual buildup to the full correction helping the patient adapt more comfortably.[25, 28] This prevents a potential sudden dramatic substantial size difference (aniseikonia) between the images seen between the two eyes. An extreme example would be if the patient was aphakic in only one eye. Except for possible traumatic cases with a resultant cataract and secondary intraocular structural compromise, today all adult patients would receive an intraocular lens implant after routine surgical cataract removal, essentially eliminating the risk for anisometropia. On the other hand, unilateral congenital cataracts do occur in infants and very young children that could result in only one cataract being removed and the patient being too young for an intraocular lens implant. This would result in substantial anisometropia between the two eyes. Contact lenses often work well in these cases since they provide an optical correction with minimal image size disparity between the eyes.

Most adults who have small amounts of anisometropia can tolerate wearing spectacles. Those who have larger differences in image size from the prismatic effects usually experience this only when viewing objects through the peripheral sections of the spectacle ophthalmic lens. These patients should be instructed to turn their head, instead of their eyes, when looking at an object that is to their side.[28]

Various other ophthalmic lens modifications may help alleviate or minimize the image disparity. Maintaining the same lens base curve as what was in their previous habitual spectacles often helps.[28] The optical centers of the spectacle lenses should align with the eyes. Incorrect centration often induces undesirable prism, resulting in enhanced anisophoria. Make sure that the vertex distance from the spectacle lens to the eye remains consistent to the patient's previous habitual correction. This is most critical in refractive errors over 4.00 diopters since a change in the vertex distance will result in an incorrect final dioptric power. A change in the ophthalmic lens material such as plastic to glass can adjust for peripheral lens thickness and minimize the prismatic effect, especially in high myopic prescriptions. Plastic lens material is frequently one-third thicker than glass lens material which has a higher index of refraction. Finally, in cases of prism effect being induced in the vertical meridian and causing diplopia when the patient looks down to read, slab-off prism is required to enable comfortable use of a bifocal or multifocal.[24, 28]

Besides the above-discussed refractive issues that can cause altered size, shape and tilt illusions, retinal pathology in the area of the macula can also cause such illusions. These patients may have retinal metamorphopsia, retinal micropsia, or retinal macropsia. Refer to the Metamorphopsia section of Chapter 7 for a more in-depth discussion of these macular structural changes.

Altered Color

For a detailed explanation of chromatopsia and all the various color aberrations, see Chapter 7. Here we will discuss briefly the three most frequent color illusion aberrations.

There are three principal image color changes that patients may experience during an illusion: erythropsia, brunescence, and cyanopsia. Erythropsia, or red-tinted vision, has the smallest differential and is almost always related to hemorrhage somewhere in the eye. Typically, this hemorrhage is found in the vitreous, but it has also been seen with intraretinal hemorrhage.[29]

There are two main causes of brunescence, which is the yellowing of perception: digoxin toxicity and cataracts. Digoxin toxicity has been traditionally associated with yellowing of the vision and has been reported to cause yellow floaters.[30, 31] However, digoxin induced brunescence has also been seen in patients with therapeutic digoxin levels.[2]

Cataract is the second common cause of brunescence. As the cataract progresses, the natural lens develops the yellow-brown coloration, called brunescence, which dulls the vibrancy of all the other visible colors.[32] This process is very slow as it occurs over the lifetime but culminates in the typical symptoms of blurry vision, haze, and glare due to bright lights. It can eventually lead to white objects being perceived as having a yellow-brown tone to them. Interestingly, since this occurs so slowly over the patient's lifetime, they may not notice this change in color perception. That is, until they have the cataracts removed and very rapidly their color perception goes back to "normal." This leads to a different kind of altered color perception called cyanopsia.[32]

Cyanopsia is a blue discoloration of the vision. The most common cause of this color aberration occurs immediately after undergoing cataract removal.[33] One theory for this is that after removing the cataract, patients rapidly regain their color vision, meaning that they are now more aware of the perception of blue color since the blue light was filtered out by the brunescent cataract over many years.[32] Further support for this theory is seen in a study where yellow intraocular lenses were implanted during cataract surgery and these patients reported cyanopsia less frequently than patients who received clear intraocular lens implants.[34, 35] This illusion is typically transient as the patients eventually get accustomed to their new perception of overall improved color. Other causes of cyanopsia include side effects of medications such as sildenafil or ethionamide.[36, 37]

The eye exhibits both spherical and chromatic aberrations. Spherical aberration occurs because of paraxial (central) and peripheral light rays focusing on different points.[13] Since the pupil acts to limit the number of light rays entering the eye, especially the peripheral light rays, spherical aberration is not an ophthalmic problem.[13] Otherwise, spherical aberration would degrade the quality of the retinal image. Chromatic aberration is induced by the prismatic

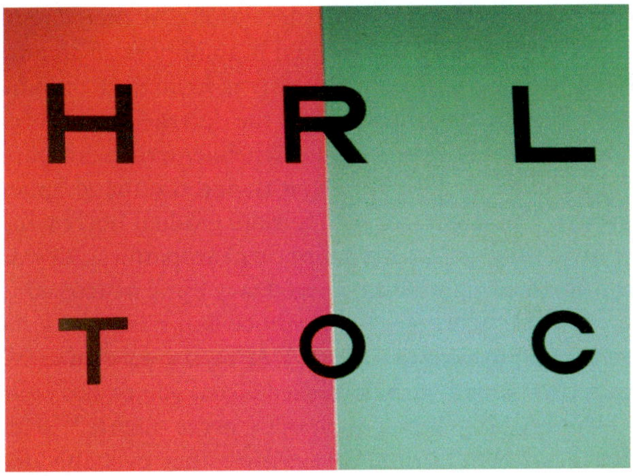

Figure 5.3 Duochrome, bichrome, or red-green test.

qualities of the natural lens. The eye generally focuses on an object at some midpoint in the visible color spectrum such as yellow. More practically, this color aberration can be used to our clinical advantage when refining the final spherical spectacle refraction. The specific test is known as the duochrome, bichrome, or red-green test (Figure 5.3). In a standard white light subjective refraction, ophthalmic lens dioptric powers are measured to correct the eye for a wavelength near the middle of the visible spectrum.[3] This test is done as a monocular test. To perform this test, simultaneously present both a green and a red target to the patient on the eyechart by using colored filters in the acuity projector. These two colors lie on either side of the bisected eyechart and equidistant by dioptrically equal amounts from the midpoint color (yellow).[3, 25] The patient sees black letters against a green background on one side and a red background on the other side of the eyechart.[3] If the eye has residual myopia, the letters of the eyechart will appear clearer on the red side and a minus sphere must be added in the phoropter (in –0.25 diopter increments) until the letters on the red and green halves are equally black and distinct.[3, 25] On the other hand, if the eye has residual hyperopia, the letters of the eyechart will appear clearer on the green side and a plus sphere must be added in the phoropter (in +0.25 diopter increments).[3, 25] Once the endpoint of equality of letter clarity in both red and green sides is reached, the red and green focal points are dioptrically equidistant from the retina and an optimal refraction has been achieved.

Decreased Brightness

Some patients may complain of seeing one image as being dimmer than the other when comparing between the eyes. This is typically caused by optic neuropathy in the eye that sees the "dimmer" image. Their description can be either decreased brightness (dim) or less vivid colors (dull). As there are many causes of optic neuropathy, limiting the differential is an important step in establishing the underlying etiology. One common way is to analyze the time period that the onset of visual changes occurred. If the decrease in brightness came on rapidly, pathologies such as optic neuritis, ischemic optic neuropathy, inflammatory (non-demyelinating) optic neuropathy, and traumatic optic neuropathy should be suspected. This contrasts with a more gradual onset which points toward compressive or toxic/nutritional optic neuropathies. An even longer time of onset points toward compressive or hereditary optic neuropathies.[38] A key diagnostic point of optic neuritis is the presence of a relative afferent pupillary defect (RAPD) on physical exam.[38, 39] RAPD, also known as Marcus Gunn pupil, is always accompanied with decreased visual acuity and color vision loss (especially the color red) in patients with optic nerve disease.[40] If a patient has diminished visual acuity but normal color vision, they probably do not have optic nerve disease. The swinging flashlight test is performed to test for a RAPD. In this test the light from a transilluminator or penlight is directed first into one pupil, then moved over quickly to the other pupil, and this is repeated several times while both pupils' response is observed.[40] The test is done in a dimly lit room, with the patient gazing at distance and not at the light source.[40] By allowing 3 to 5 seconds of illumination on each side, a RAPD can be identified in the pupil that becomes paradoxically larger when the light is directed to the involved side.[40] The RAPD can be measured subjectively or objectively by using neutral density filters which are held in front of the uninvolved eye and progressively increasing the filter density until the pupil reactions on the swing test are equal.[40]

Occasionally a clinician who is examining a patient at the hospital bedside or does not have access to an optical coherence tomography scanner in the clinic may need to distinguish between subtle unilateral macular disease and retrobulbar optic neuropathy. The photo-stress recovery test (glare recovery test, macular dazzle test) is a rapid and uncomplicated clinical test that is effective in distinguishing the vision loss seen in these two different ophthalmic pathologies. This test is based on the principle that visual pigments bleach when exposed to an intense light source, resulting in a temporary state of sensitivity loss and reduced central visual acuity.[41] Recovery of the retinal sensitivity is dependent upon regeneration of the visual pigments.[41] A prolonged recovery time (delay in the regeneration of the visual pigments) following light stimulation of the retina/macula will be present if there is disease in the choriocapillaris, retinal pigment epithelium, and outer retinal layers.[42, 43] In a normal eye, or in an eye with optic neuropathy, the recovery time should be 50 seconds or less while in an eye that has retinal/macular disease the recovery is greatly prolonged (90 to 180 seconds).[42, 43] In central serous retinopathy, recovery can take several minutes. The photo-stress recovery test is performed by determining the patient's best-corrected visual acuity, covering one eye with an opaque occluder and then having the patient look directly at a bright focal light source such as a transilluminator or penlight that is held 2 to 3 cm in front of the unoccluded eye for 10 seconds.[41–43] The time needed for the patient to be able to read to within one line of their best-corrected visual acuity is recorded and is known as the photo-stress recovery time.[41–43]

It may also be necessary to distinguish between optic neuropathy and amblyopia in a patient with long-standing vision loss in one eye. In such cases a 2-log unit neutral density filter (Kodak Wratten 2, No. 96, ND 2.00) should be used.[43, 44] The use of such a neutral density filter in healthy eyes reduces the visual acuity by approximately two lines (e.g., from 20/20 to 20/40), while in eyes with mild strabismic amblyopia, vision is only slightly reduced, stays the same, or actually improves.[43, 44] With an optic nerve conduction defect such as retrobulbar optic neuritis, vision usually is reduced drastically when a neutral density filter is placed before the involved eye (e.g., from 20/60 to 20/200 or 20/400).[43]

Another possibility for the decrease in brightness could be a dense anterior chamber hemorrhage (hyphema) or a vitreous hemorrhage (Figure 5.4).[10] In contrast to the previous cause of decreased brightness, which was due to optic nerve dysfunction, this part of the differential is due to dense fluids (hemorrhage) which absorb the light before it reaches the retina. Patients with vitreous hemorrhages often also complain of dark floaters. A corneal scar or cataract would not cause these symptoms as these pathologies cause a scattering of light rather than absorbing it.[10]

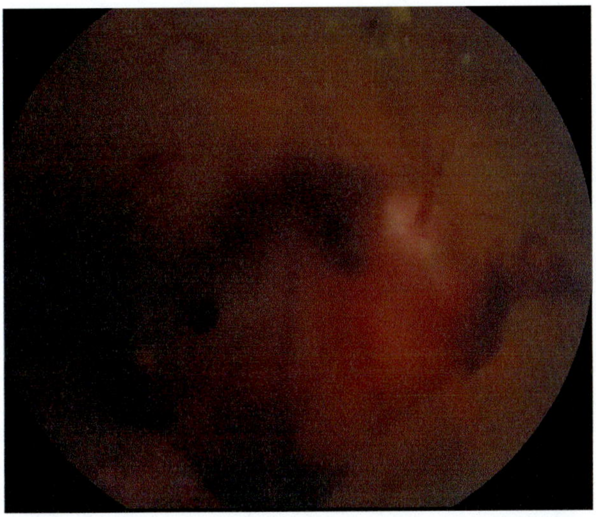

Figure 5.4 Vitreous hemorrhages as typically seen in patients with proliferative diabetic retinopathy. The optic disc is viewed as a "headlight in the fog".

Altered Motion

The most well-known alteration of motion is the Pulfrich stereo-illusion, where patients falsely view a pendulum as swinging in an ellipsoid or circular excursion (3-dimensional motion) rather than along the actual plane perpendicular to their direction of view (visual axis) (2-dimensional motion) (Figure 5.5).[41, 45]

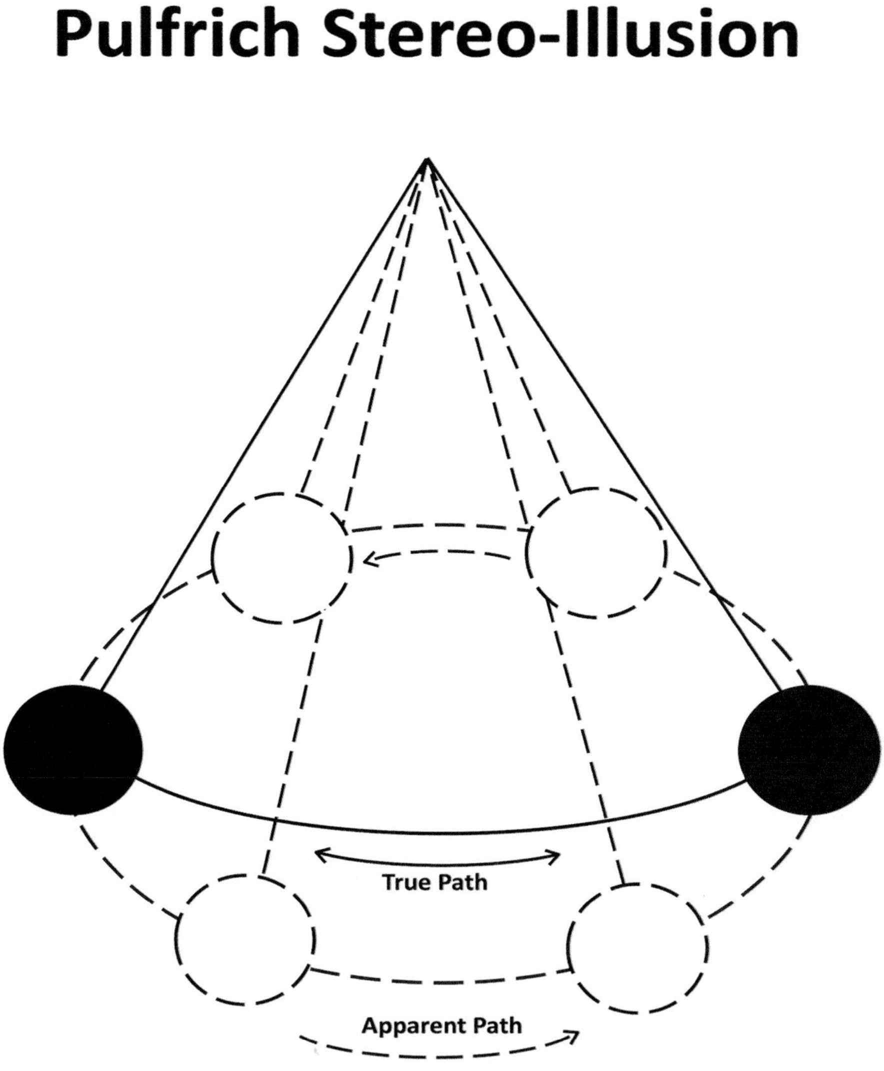

Figure 5.5 Pulfrich stereo-illusion. A pendulum appears to be swinging in an ellipsoid or circular excursion (3-dimensional motion) rather than along the actual true single plane perpendicular to the visual axis (2-dimensional motion). Both eyes must be open simultaneously to visualize this illusion. In this example, the right eye has a slower optic nerve signal conduction than the left eye. The patient perceives the pendulum swinging in a counterclockwise direction.

This illusion is due to a lapse in the optic nerve signal conduction between the two eyes. When one eye has a slower optic nerve conduction, say the left eye, then the patient will perceive the pendulum swinging in a clockwise direction.[41, 46] If there is a conduction deficit in the optic nerve of the right eye, the rotation will appear counterclockwise.[41, 46] Although there is no definitive diagnostic criteria for the Pulfrich phenomenon, one possible way to test for it is to create a pendulum and assess what the patient sees when the pendulum is swung along a 2-dimentional plane.[47] Patients who experience this motion stereo-illusion can have difficulties with driving a car, walking over uneven terrain, or participating in sports such as softball, baseball, volleyball, pickleball and tennis.[41] There is no definitive treatment for patients who experience the Pulfrich phenomenon. However, one study found that by placing a light filter over the "good" eye could partially equalize the latency between nerve signals and relieve some of the symptoms.[47] This result wasn't seen in all patients tested; however, the authors of this study concluded that since it is a relatively inexpensive treatment that it should be tried in patients with the Pulfrich phenomenon.[47] The Pulfrich illusion is a useful companion test for color vision evaluation, pupillary testing for RAPD, photostress recovery testing, and brightness sensation measurement.

Another form of altered motion is oscillopsia where patients perceive stationary objects as moving. This is most commonly seen in patients with large amplitude nystagmus.[10] During the nystagmus beating, the eyes produce multiple "pictures" on the retina which the brain then interprets as movement.[48] It should be noted that patients with congenital nystagmus do not perceive this movement.[48] Another cause of oscillopsia is a defective vestibulo-ocular reflex.[10] This reflex is typically used to maintain a clear picture while the head or body is moving. When this is defective, it causes a similar situation to nystagmus where multiple images are projected onto the retina, causing a blurring of vision or a perception of motion when there is none.[49] One way to test for a vestibulo-ocular reflex defect is by having the patient read a Snellen near card while rapidly moving the head side to side.[10] This will cause a decrease in at least two lines on the near point card chart.[10] Currently, there is no effective treatment for vestibulo-ocular reflex defects.[49]

Illustrative Case

A 23-year-old white female noticed a sudden severe loss of vision in her right eye. Her only accompanying symptom was pain with eye movement. She never had any previous eye problems and did not wear glasses or contact lenses. Her last routine eye examination by her optometrist, approximately one year earlier, was unremarkable. She denied any other systemic or neurologic symptoms and was on no medication. She did not smoke or use illicit drugs.

Her uncorrected vision in the right eye (OD) was counting fingers at 3 feet and 20/20 in the left eye (OS). There was no improvement with pinhole testing, OD. The patient had a 4+ RAPD OD and although her extraocular motility was normal; she felt pain in and behind her OD with these ocular excursions. She failed the Ishihara color test only in the OD. Red-cap desaturation testing was

0% OD and 100% OS. The slit-lamp evaluation was normal, as were her intraocular pressures. A formal computerized visual field showed dramatic overall depression with central field loss OD and a normal visual field OS (Figure 5.6). A dilated fundus examination showed only mild disc edema OD (Figure 5.7). The OS fundus examination was normal.

The patient had a typical optic neuritis presentation. As per the Optic Neuritis Treatment Trial (ONTT), magnetic resonance imagining of the brain and orbits

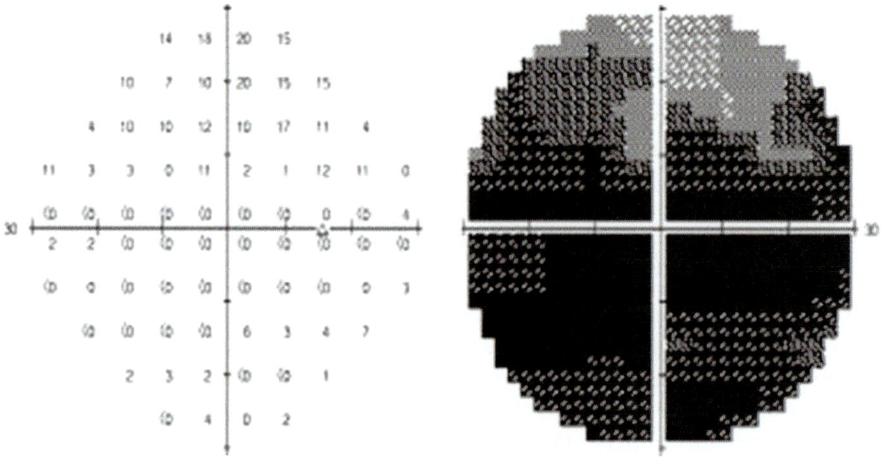

Figure 5.6 Formal computerized visual field showed dramatic overall depression with central field loss in right eye.

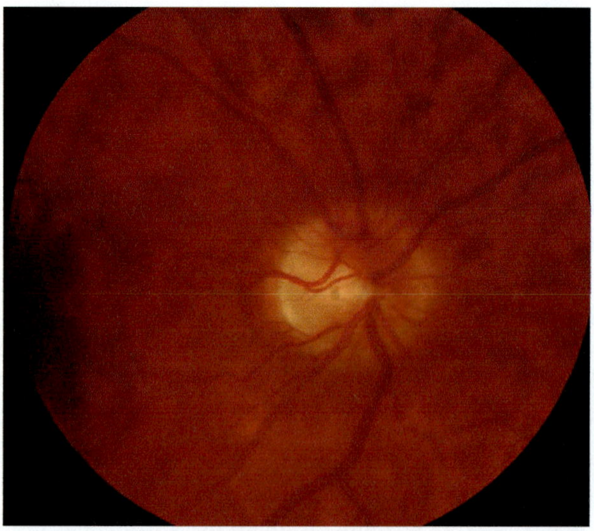

Figure 5.7 Mild disc edema in right eye.

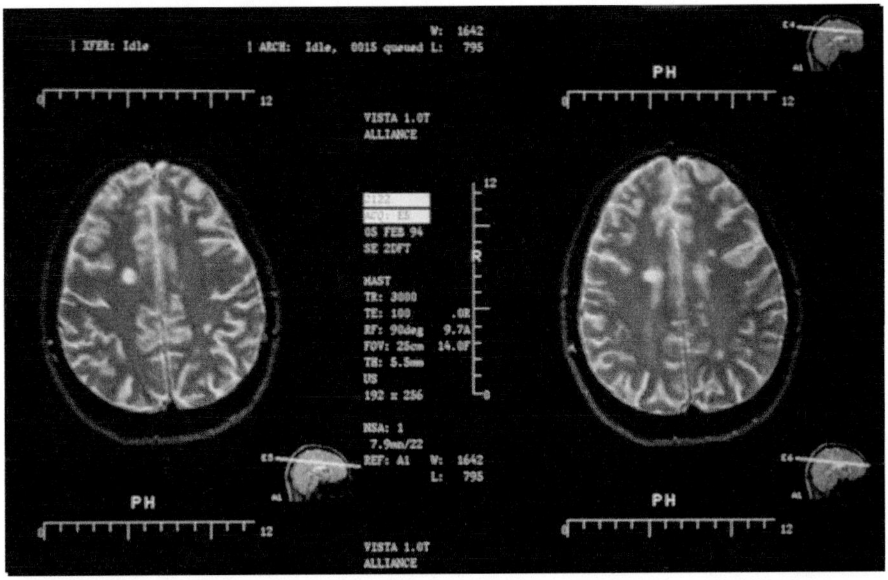

Figure 5.8 Magnetic resonance imaging showing multiple images of several periventricular white matter lesions which are characteristic findings of demyelinating disease (plaques seen as bright areas).

was obtained.[50] It showed multiple periventricular white matter lesions which are characteristic findings of demyelinating disease (Figure 5.8). The patient was started on intravenous methylprednisolone for three days, followed by 11 days of oral prednisone as per the ONTT protocol.[51] Either no treatment or treatment with intravenous corticosteroid therapy followed by an oral corticosteroid taper is appropriate; intravenous corticosteroids may benefit the patient in terms of faster recovery to normal vision which is what this patient desired.[52] In the ONTT, oral corticosteroid therapy alone was found to be associated with an increase in the rate of new episodes of optic neuritis. Oral prednisone therapy alone without starting intravenous steroid treatment first, should not be initiated.[51]The patient was also referred to a neurologist for additional evaluation of her probable demyelinating disease.

REFERENCES

1. The Beatles, *We Can Work It Out.* Capitol Records. Written by John Lennon and Paul McCartney.
2. Butler Jr VP, et al., Digitalis-induced visual disturbances with therapeutic serum digitalis concentrations. *Ann Intern Med.* 1995;123(9):676–80.
3. Goss DA, et al., *Introduction to the Optics of the Eye.* Woburn, MA: Butterworth-Heinemann; 2002: 1–39 and 155–77.

4. McCready D, *The Moon illusion Explained*. https://www.uww.edu/Documents/colleges/cls/Departments/Psychology/Mccread_Moon_Illusions.pdf. Accessed June 21, 2025.
5. Kaufman L, et al., Explaining the moon illusion. *Proc Natl Acad Sci.* 2000;97(1):500–5.
6. New World Encyclopedia, *Müller-Lyer Illusion*. https://www.newworldencyclopedia.org/entry/Muller-Lyer_illusion. Accessed June 21, 2025.
7. Luckiesh M, *Visual Illusions: Their Causes, Characteristics & Applications*. New York: Dover Publishers; 1965: 76–101.
8. Sheth T, *BMJ*. 2024. https://doi.org/10.1136/bmj-2023-076413.
9. Williams DR, Nonoptical and accessory devices. In: Brilliant RL, ed, *Essentials of Low Vision Practice*. Boston: Butterworth-Heinemann; 1999: 269–90.
10. Burde RM, et al., *Clinical Decisions in Neuro-Ophthalmology*, 3rd edn. St. Louis: Mosby; 2002: 114–35.
11. Palmieri GR, et al., *Eur J Case Rep Intern Med*. 2021.
12. Graf M, et al., How to deal with diplopia. *Rev Neurol (Paris)*. 2012;168(10):720–8.
13. Dowaliby M, *Practical Aspects of Ophthalmic Optics*, 4th edn. Boston: Butterworth-Heinemann; 2001: 1–34.
14. Hersh LA, et al., Low vision distance systems I: Spectacles and contact lenses. In: Brilliant RL, ed, *Essentials of Low Vision Practice*. Boston: Butterworth-Heinemann; 1999: 131–46.
15. Iliescu DA, et al., Management of diplopia. *Rom J Ophthalmol.* 2017;61(3):166–70.
16. Skorin L, et al., Dragged fovea diplopia syndrome after epiretinal membrane peel surgery. *Clin Surg Ophthalmol.* 2013;31(1):12–7.
17. Yau GSK, et al., Unilateral papilledema and choroidal folds: an uncommon presentation of idiopathic intracranial hypertension. *Sur Curr Res.* 2014;04(04):1–3.
18. Morris RJ, Double vision as a presenting symptom in an ophthalmic casualty department. *Eye.* 1991;5(1):124–9.
19. Comer RM, et al., Causes and outcomes for patients presenting with diplopia to an eye casualty department. *Eye.* 2007;21(3):413–8.
20. Danchaivijetr C, et al., Diplopia and eye movement disorders. *J Neurol Neurosurg Psychiatry.* 2004;75(Suppl 4):iv24–iv31.
21. Barton JJS, et al., Disorders of higher function. In: Kline LB, Foroozan R, eds, *Neuro-Ophthalmology: Review Manual*, 7th edn. Thorofare, NJ: SLACK Incorp; 2013: 245–56.
22. Chu YR, et al., Corneal cross-linking. In: Freisberg L, Lighthizer N, Skorin L, et al, eds, *The Ophthalmic Laser Handbook*. Philadelphia: Wolters Kluwer; 2022: 165–75.
23. Werner DL, Press LJ, *Clinical Pearls in Refractive Care*. Boston: Butterworth-Heinemann; 2002: 181–219.

24. Rosenfeld M, Refractive status of the eye. In: Benjamin WJ, ed, *Borish's Clinical Refraction*. Philadelphia: Saunders; 1998: 10.
25. Michaels DD, *Visual Optics and Refraction: A Clinical Approach*, 3rd edn. St. Louis: C. V. Mosby Co.; 1985: 316–34 and 484–505.
26. Remole A, Anisophoria and aniseikonia: Part I. The relation between optical anisophoria and aniseikonia. *Am J Optom Physiol Opt.* 1989;66:659–70.
27. Remole A, Anisophoria and aniseikonia: Part II. The management of optical anisophoria. *Am J Optom Physiol Opt.* 1989;66:736–46.
28. Michaels DD, *Anisometropia*. Bowie, MD: The National Academy of Opticianry; 1988: 1–17.
29. Vaphiades MS, et al., Erythropsia and chromatopsia: Case study and brief review. *Neuro-Ophthalmology.* 2021;45(1):56–60.
30. Arnold WN, Loftus LS, Xanthopsia and van Gogh's yellow palette. *Eye.* 1991;5(5):503–10.
31. Shi L, et al., Colored floaters as a manifestation of digoxin toxicity. *Am J Ophthalmol Case Reports.* 2018;10:233–5.
32. Pollock JL, et al., Vision, knowledge, and the mystery link. *Philosophical Perspectives.* 2005;19:309–51.
33. Kitakawa T, et al., Evaluation of early state of cyanopsia with subjective color settings immediately after cataract removal surgery. *J Opt Soc Am.* 2009;26(6):1375–81.
34. Yuan Z, et al., Contrast sensitivity and color vision with a yellow intraocular lens. *Am J Ophthalmol.* 2004;138(1):138–40.
35. Hayashi K, et al., Visual function in patients with yellow tinted intraocular lenses compared with vision in patients with non-tinted intraocular lenses. *Br J Ophthalmol.* 2006;90(8):1019–23.
36. Lee CH, et al., A case report of cyanopsia after taking sildenafil. *Kor J Clin Pharm.* 2020;30(1):59–64.
37. Jain AK, et al., Ethionamide induced blue vision (cyanopsia): Case report. *Ind J Tuberculosis.* 2020;67(3):333–5.
38. Behbehani R, Clinical approach to optic neuropathies. *Clin Ophthalmol.* 2007;1(3):233–46.
39. Skorin L, Optic neuritis. In: Onofrey BE, Skorin L, Holdeman NR, eds, *Ocular Therapeutics Handbook: A Clinical Manual*, 4th edn. Philadelphia: Wolters Kluwer; 2020: 626–8.
40. Skorin L, et al., Pupil abnormalities. In: Onofrey BE, Skorin L, Holdeman NR, eds, *Ocular Therapeutics Handbook: A Clinical Manual*, 4th edn. Philadelphia: Wolters Kluwer; 2020: 578–80.
41. Wall M, et al., Principles and techniques of the examination of the visual sensory system. In: Miller NR, Newman NJ, eds, *Walsh & Hoyt's Clinical Neuro-Ophthalmology*, 6th edn. Philadelphia: Lippincott Wiliams & Wilkins; 2005: 83–149.
42. Glaser JS, et al., The photostress recovery testing in the clinical assessment of visual function. *Am J Ophthalmol.* 1977;83:255–60.

43. Glaser JS, et al., Neuro-ophthalmologic examination: The visual sensory system. In: Glaser JS, ed, *Neuro-ophthalmology*, 2nd edn. Philadelphia: J. B. Lippincott Co.; 1990: 9–36.
44. Von Noorden GK, et al., Visual acuity in normal and amblyopic patients under reduced illumination: 1. Behavior of visual acuity with and without neutral density filter. *Arch Ophthalmol.* 1959;61(4):533–5.
45. Pulfrich C, Die Stereoskopie im Dienste der isochromen und heterochromen Photometrie. *Naturwissenschaften.* 1922;10:553–64.
46. Qian N, et al., A physiological model for motion-stereo integration and a unified explanation of Pulfrich-like phenomena. *Vis Res.* 1997;37(12):1683–98.
47. Farr J, et al., The Pulfrich phenomenon: practical implications of the assessment of cases and effectiveness of treatment. *Neuro-Ophthalmology.* 2018;42(6):349–55.
48. Straube A, Bronstein A, Straumann D, Nystagmus and oscillopsia. *Eur J Neurol.* 2012;19(1):6–14.
49. Swain SK, et al., Vestibulo-ocular reflex–A narrative review. *Matrix Sci Med.* 2023;7(4):90–4.
50. Dogahe SJ, et al., Acute optic neuritis: An update on approach and management. *Ophthalmic Vis Res.* 2023;18(4):433–40.
51. Beck RW, et al., A randomized controlled trial of corticosteroids in the treatment of acute optic neuritis. The Optic Neuritis Study Group. *New Eng J Med.* 1992;326(9):581–8.
52. Gal RL, et al., *Cochrane Database Syst Rev.* 2015.

Chapter 6

BINOCULAR HEMIFIELD ILLUSIONS

Jesse Britt and Leonid Skorin, Jr.

Introduction

"Seeing is deceiving.[1]"

— Matthew Luckiesh

In contrast to hallucinations, illusions are false perceptions of visual stimuli that disappear with eye closure.[2] An illusion does not generally exist physically.[1] These illusions can be either monocular or binocular. Binocular illusions can be further differentiated into full-field or hemifield defects. Binocular full-field illusions have been discussed previously in Chapter 5. This chapter will focus on binocular hemifield illusions, the various etiologies causing them, and the associated visual alterations. Primarily, binocular hemifield illusions are caused by (1) occipitoparietotemporal lesions, (2) vertebrobasilar transient ischemic attacks (TIA) and, rarely, (3) migraine.

Occipitoparietotemporal Lesions

Illusions and hallucinations caused by occipitoparietotemporal lesions are often unilateral, confined to a certain hemifield, and have a concomitant hemianopsia. These lesions can be due to infarct (stroke), tumor, inflammation, dysplasia, or rarely arteriovenous malformations. Illusions and hallucinations caused by lesions to the posterior cerebrum can be intermittent, transient, or persistent.[3]

Prior to neuroimaging and assisting in localizing any such intracranial lesion, a formal visual field evaluation should be performed. The visual pathway extends like a roadway from the retina in the back of the eye to the occipital pole of the brain. Any interruption of this roadway results in a visual field defect. The specific characteristics of the defect often lend clues to the location of an underlying intracranial lesion. The three general defects seen on a visual field include: (1) Contraction, an absolute field loss; (2) Depression, reduced sensitivity to light without an actual loss of field; and (3) Scotoma, a partial or complete defect surrounded by a normal field of vision. A field defect in only one eye suggests a possible lesion anterior to the optic chiasm. Binocular defects may originate from the optic chiasm, optic tracts, optic radiations or visual cortex. The latter three would encompass the occipitoparietotemporal regions.

Congruity refers to the similarity between binocular visual field defects. Dissimilar field defects occur in lesions of the optic tract or in both optic nerves.

DOI: 10.1201/9781003633365-6

More congruous field defects result from lesions involving the optic radiations and visual cortex.

The density or severity of visual field loss in many cases reflects its etiology. A vascular etiology such as a stroke causes an extremely dense defect. Slowly growing tumors produce less severe defects.

The slope is an additional characteristic of field defects that offer diagnostic value. The slope defines the margins of the field defect and reflects the degree of change. For example, a gentle slope, marking the margin between a more severe and milder defect, suggests that the underlying lesion is still changing—whether progressing or improving. A steep slope would imply a stable lesion, such as a previous old injury or stroke.

Encompassing all these characteristics confirms that the shape of the presenting visual field defect gives the clinician significant diagnostic value and helps guide the neuroradiological imaging.

Lesions of the retina and optic nerve cause monocular defects and always exhibit a relative afferent pupillary defect on that same side (see Illustrative Case 1). Lesions that impinge or damage the body of the chiasm produce bitemporal hemianopsia (see Illustrative Case 2). Lesions located posterior to the chiasm produce homonymous hemianopic visual field defects—defects that occur on the same side in both eyes and respect the vertical meridian.[4] Optic tract lesions result in homonymous, yet incongruous, field defects. Lesions of the optic tract can result in a relative afferent pupillary defect contralateral to the side of the brain lesion. Lesions affecting the optic radiations produce bilateral field defects that are more congruous than optic tract lesions with increasing congruity the more posterior the lesion is located in the brain.[5] The fibers of the optic radiations that correspond to the inferior retina spread out in Meyer's loop through the temporal lobe in the brain and result in superior homonymous visual field defects, or at least defects that are denser above the horizontal meridian (Figures 6.1a, b).[5] Temporal lobe dysfunction usually produces formed hallucinations.[6] Temporal lobe damage may also cause aphasia, memory deficits, and auditory hallucinations. The fibers of the optic radiations that correspond to the superior retina wind through the parietal lobe and create homonymous inferior visual field defects such as quadrantanopsias that are denser below than above (Figures 6.2a, b).[5] These tend to be more congruous than the defects associated with temporal lobe lesions. Because the parietal lobe is predominantly concerned with sensory modalities, many lesions in this region cause sensory deficits or hemifield neglect if the nondominant hemisphere is damaged. The occurring visual symptoms include photopsias, metamorphopsia, difficulty with color vision, illusions, and hallucinations.[4] These latter phenomena tend to occur in the defective portion of the visual field.[4]

All fibers from the optic radiations converge at the visual cortex along the calcarine fissure. The posterior occipital lobe tip and 40% to 50% of the contiguous mesial (midline) surface of the occipital lobes are devoted to central (macular)

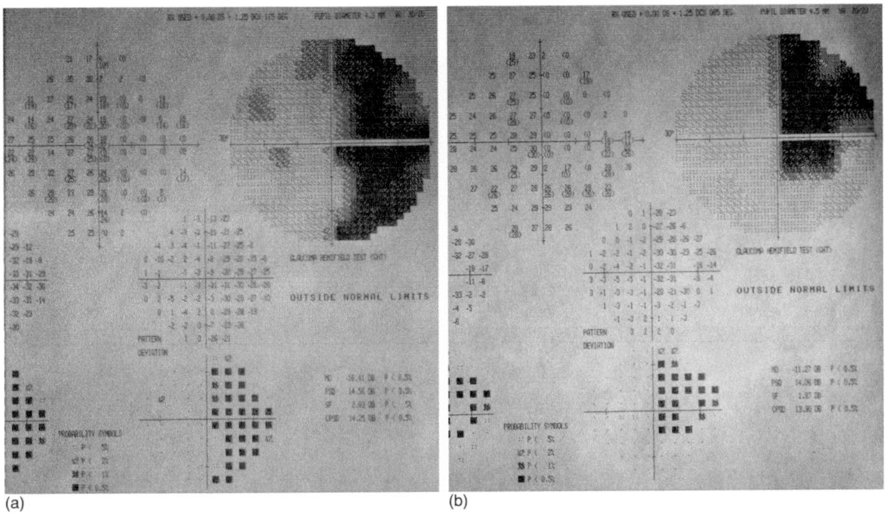

Figure 6.1 (a) Left eye - right homonymous incongruous hemianopsia. (b) Right eye – right homonymous incongruous hemianopsia denser superiorly, suggesting left optic tract - anterior temporal lobe involvement. A superior congruous homonymous quadrantanopsia is usually diagnostic for lesions in the temporal lobe but may also occur from a lesion of the inferior lip of the calcarine fissure in the occipital lobe.

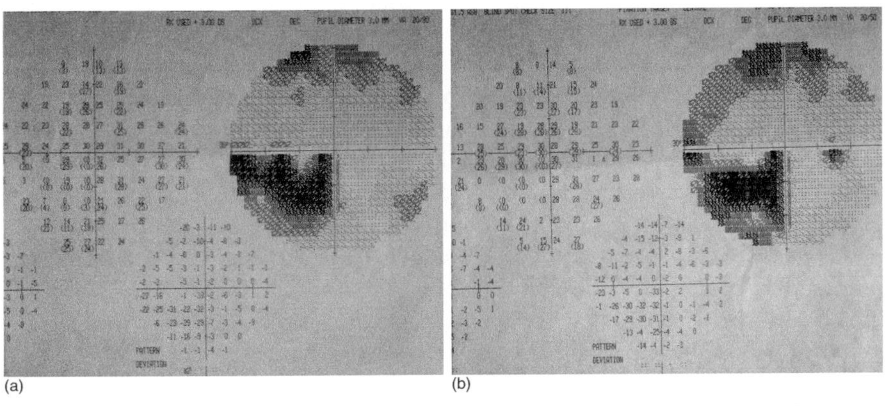

Figure 6.2 (a) Left eye – left inferior homonymous congruous quandrantanopsia. (b) Right eye – left inferior homonymous congruous quadrantanopsia, suggesting a focal lesion, in this case an infarction, in the right parietal lobe or the upper lip of the calcarine fissure in the occipital lobe.

vision while the anterior end corresponds to the peripheral field.[5] Occipital lobe lesions produce visual field defects that are homonymous and highly congruous.[5] Homonymous hemianopsia is often highly disabling for patients, causing problems with reading and visual scanning due to the patient's inability to scan into the blind field. These patients cannot legally drive in most states in

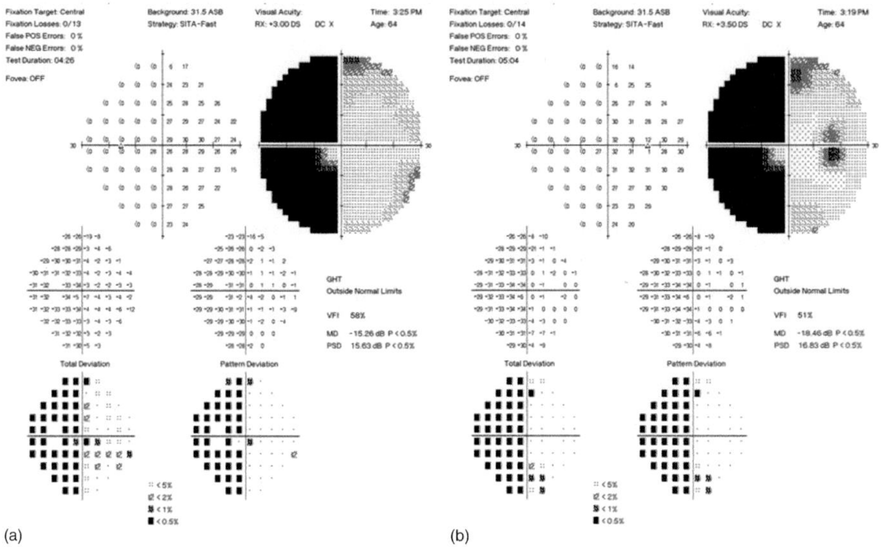

Figure 6.3 (a) Left eye – Left homonymous hemianopsia with macular sparing. (b) Right eye – Left homonymous hemianopsia with macular sparing.

the United States, resulting in significant consequences for their vocational and personal lives. Clinically, patients with homonymous hemianopsia may—or may not—be aware of their visual field loss since they will have no other neurologic symptoms other than visual field loss. In addition, visual acuity is preserved in most cases, especially if their visual field defect exhibits macular sparing. Macular sparing is another clinical feature of these lesions and refers to the tendency of occipital lesions to produce homonymous visual fields that spare the central 5 degrees of the visual field (Figures 6.3a,b).[5] This helps localize such a visual field defect with macula sparing to a lesion in the visual cortex. Macular sparing may be due to the occipital poles receiving a dual blood supply from branches of the posterior cerebral and middle cerebral arteries.[5,7] If there is a lesion, most usually the result of an infarction, at the tip of the occipital lobe, the resulting visual scotomatous defect would be a homonymous congruent quadrantanopsia located centrally in the macular field (Figures 6.4a–c).

There have been several models designed to try and explain how illusions and hallucinations form due to these lesions.[8] Of these, the three models that carry the most validity are: (1) the release phenomena whereby disrupted visual input causes atypical central processing that leads to altered perception, (2) the presence of localized seizure activity at or near the lesion, and (3) the development of migraine aura activity caused by the lesion.

For the release phenomena model, it has been proposed that the lesions spare the visual association cortex which then becomes disengaged from normal visual input by the obstructing lesion present in the primary visual cortex. Thus, lack

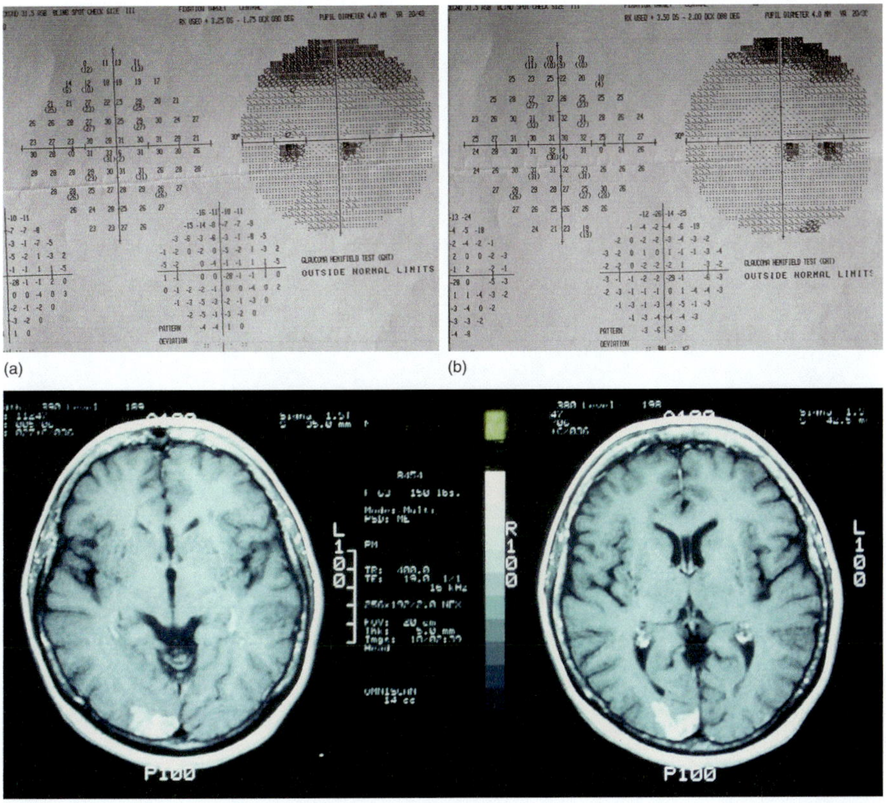

(a) (b) (c)

Figure 6.4 (a) Left eye – Right inferior homonymous congruous quadrantanopsia, central, involving macula field. (b) Right eye - Right inferior homonymous congruous quadrantanopsia, central, involving macula field. (c) Magnetic resonance imaging showing infarction in the left occipital tip, superior calcarine cortex.

of visual input from the primary visual cortex leads to disinhibition of the visual association cortex. In turn, the disinhibited visual association cortex produces images that get "released" and perceived by the individual.

In contrast to the release phenomena model, illusions and hallucinations that occur may be due to partial seizures which originate from the primary visual cortex. These illusions typically present as lines, stars, dots, zigzags, squares, circles, etc. Often these start in one hemifield and may quickly spread to encompass the entire field of vision. Identifying illusions and hallucinations due to partial seizure activity is achieved by the clinician recognizing the occurrence of specific accompanying automatisms such as staring, loss of consciousness, excessive blinking, eyelid twitching, nystagmus, or other tonic-clonic movements.

Similarly, migraine aura activity at the site of an occipitoparietotemporal lesion can also cause visual phenomena. These are typically unformed images with

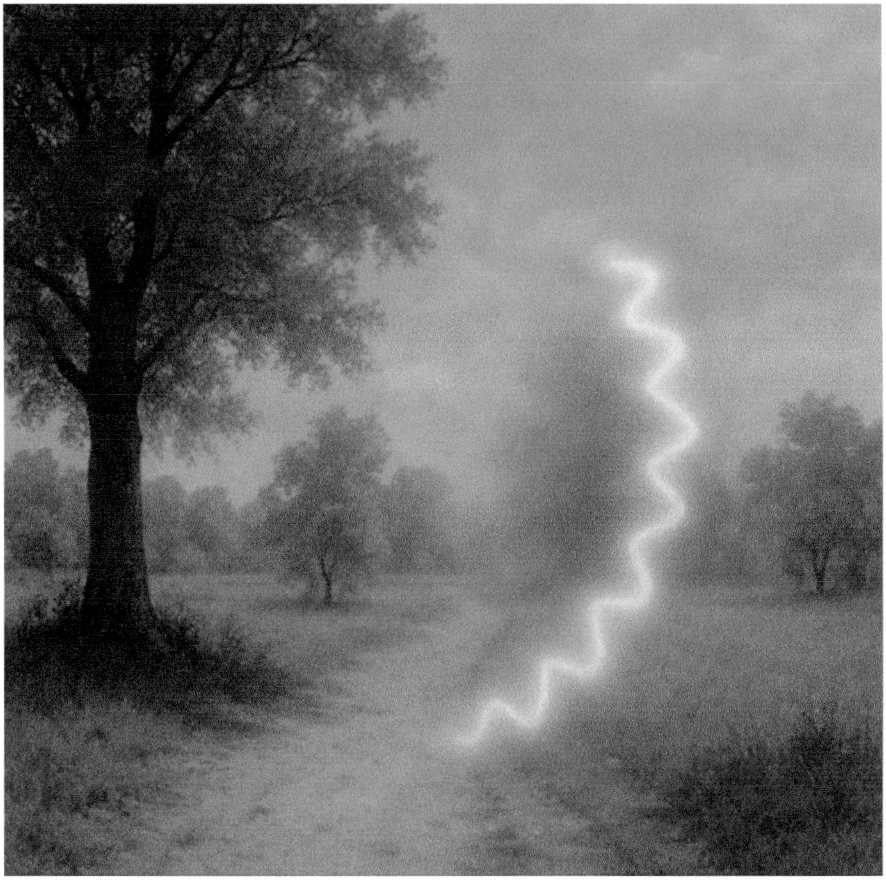

Figure 6.5 Representation of partial scintillating scotoma commonly seen with ocular migraine.

a large portion of individuals reporting a scintillating scotoma, described as a sparkling zigzag shape (Figure 6.5). This shape tends to spread, forming what is referred to as the marching scintillating scotoma, and is often not confined to a single hemifield. In these circumstances, other visual phenomena such as twinkling lights and sparking pinwheels are also common.

Vertebrobasilar Transient Ischemic Attacks

The vertebrobasilar system is comprised of paired vertebral arteries that merge to form the midline basilar artery, and distal branches including the posterior cerebral arteries.[9] The basilar artery and its branches (posterior cerebral arteries) supply the vast majority of the visual cortex.[9] Vertebrobasilar TIA tend to produce more transient visual phenomena, lasting only seconds to usually less than one minute, as opposed to more episodic and persistent visual phenomena seen with occipitoparietotemporal lesions. These brief visual episodes are described by patients as simply blurred vision or out-of-focus vision.[9] On the other hand, if the visual phenomena persist for longer than a few hours, then there will likely be an associated homonymous visual field defect and evidence of infarct on neuroimaging. After an occipital infarct, visual disturbances usually subside within a few weeks even with persistence of visual field loss.

Also, vertebrobasilar TIA rarely produces the zigzag shape or demonstrates "the march" across a hemifield that is characteristic of migraine. Instead, images seen with vertebrobasilar TIA consist of flakes, sparks, radiant light, and squiggly lines. Based on whether hypoperfusion affects one or both posterior cerebral arteries, these may be limited to a singular hemifield, or they may cover the entire visual field. This, along with other symptoms common in brainstem ischemia (i.e. disequilibrium, vertigo, nystagmus and oscillopsia, extremity weakness, nausea/vomiting, altered consciousness, numbness, drop attacks, and diplopia), can help differentiate vertebrobasilar TIA from migraine.

Migraine

A classic migraine is a headache that is preceded by an "aura." An aura is a neurologic disruption that tends to produce positive or negative visual phenomena, paresthesia, aphasia, and hemiparesis. This disturbance is transient and dissipates with resolution of the migraine. An aura will present in 25% of patients experiencing migraines and with unformed visual hallucinations being the predominant symptom.[7] As mentioned previously, migraine classically causes a "marching scintillating scotoma" but can cause other visual phenomena. This typically lasts about 20 to 40 minutes but can last up to one hour.[7] The scintillating scotoma will spread throughout this time, hence the term "marching."

Interestingly, a significant portion of individuals may experience visual symptoms of migraine aura without the following headache. This is commonly referred to as an acephalgic or dissociated migraine. In contrast to focal lesions which occur in the primary visual cortex, migraines rarely caused formed images. Migraines can also present with multiple neurologic deficits, well beyond just the visual findings. These tend to be an advancing event, starting with a scintillating scotoma, then developing a spreading paresthesia, and finally progressing to a possible aphasia. In contrast, focal lesions such as tumors or infarcts of the primary visual cortex will tend to have such neurologic deficits occurring simultaneously with the vision changes.

Types of Illusions/Hallucinations

Illusions come in all shapes and sizes. Visual phenomena can be perceived as changes in shape (i.e. cerebral metamorphopsia or illusory spread), changes in position (i.e. visual allesthesia, cerebral diplopia, and cerebral polyopia), changes in size (i.e. micropsia, macropsia, and teleopsia) which are discussed in Chapter 7, and visual perservation in time (i.e. palinopsia). This section will highlight some of the visual disturbances that patients may experience.

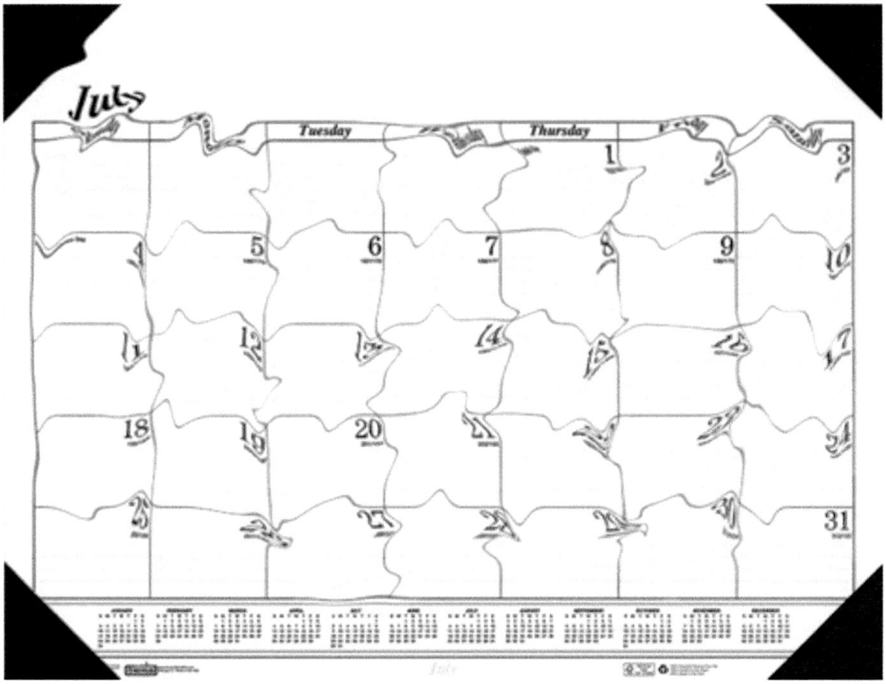

Figure 6.6 Representation of distorted vision involving the whole visual field as seen with cerebral metamorphopsia.

i. **Altered Shape**

The primary visual alteration described by patients with cerebral metamorphopsia, also known as illusory spread, results in elongations of forms and shapes in a plane with one object overlapping onto another.[7, 10] Typically, the visual scene is displaced and distorted in a disorienting manner (Figure 6.6). These visual disturbances often coincide with palinopsia or visual hallucinations. They can be intermittent or persistent, but they frequently resolve days to weeks after onset. Cerebral metamorphopsia has been described with seizures, right parietal glioma, right parietal arteriovenous malformation (distortion limited to faces), posterior cerebral infarction and even brain stem lesions.[11]

ii. **Altered Position**

Visual allesthesia is described as patients seeing the image of an object that was previously viewed as being displaced from one homonymous hemifield into the contralateral hemifield.[12, 13] For instance, an object seen to the left of fixation may be perceived moments later to the right of fixation. Patients may experience double vision (diplopia) or multiple vision - seeing multiple copies of an image at one time (polyopia) (Figure 6.7). This phenomenon is almost always associated with a homonymous hemianopia that is caused by an occipitoparietotemporal lesion present contralateral to the visual

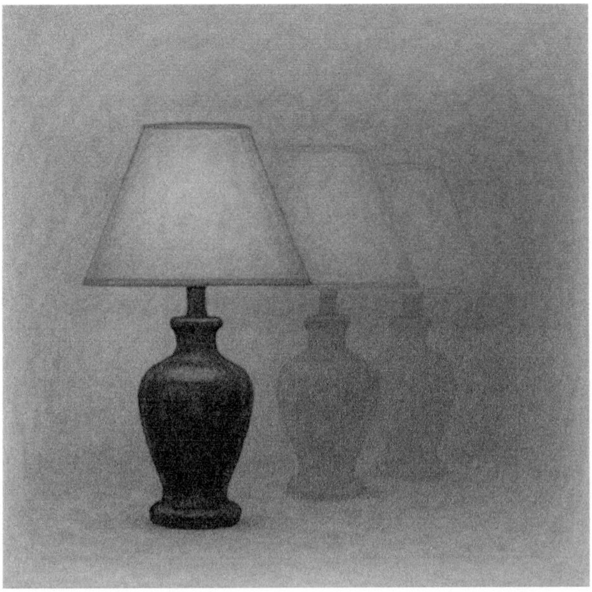

Figure 6.7 Representation of polyopia.

field deficit.[7] In one reported case, a patient with a right parieto-occipital arteriovenous malformation experienced illusory left homonymous transpositions of objects, lasting up to 15 minutes, that were originally seen in the right homonymous visual field.[12] In this case, the underlying cause was attributed to an anomalous interhemispheric transfer from a normal to an irritated parieto-occipital lobe.[12] Visual allesthesia can also occur from seizure activity.[14]

iii. Palinopsia (Palinopia, Paliopia)

Palinopsia is a form of visual perseveration in time where an image from a prior scene is "replayed" and superimposed on the patient's current field of view (Figure 6.8).[7, 9, 11, 13] Such illusions may appear discontinuous but overlapping, like multiple stroboscopic freeze-frames or a smeared "comet-tail" image of an object in motion and may be interpreted by the patient as diplopia or polyopia.[9, 13] It is thought that there are at least two forms of visual perseveration: immediate and delayed.[11] With the immediate form, an image remains even after the actual scene has passed. This immediate form is similar to the effect of experiencing "afterimages" due to prolonged or bright light exposure.[3] However, the immediate form of palinopsia typically will last up to several minutes before fading whereas the afterimage effect should only last a few seconds. With the delayed form of palinopsia, an image of a previously seen object appears after an interval of minutes to hours, sometimes repeatedly for days or even weeks.[15] The longer the image persists, it is more likely a hallucination and less likely an illusion. Although most cases of palinopsia resolve spontaneously after lasting days to weeks, some recorded cases lasted from months to years.[13, 15]

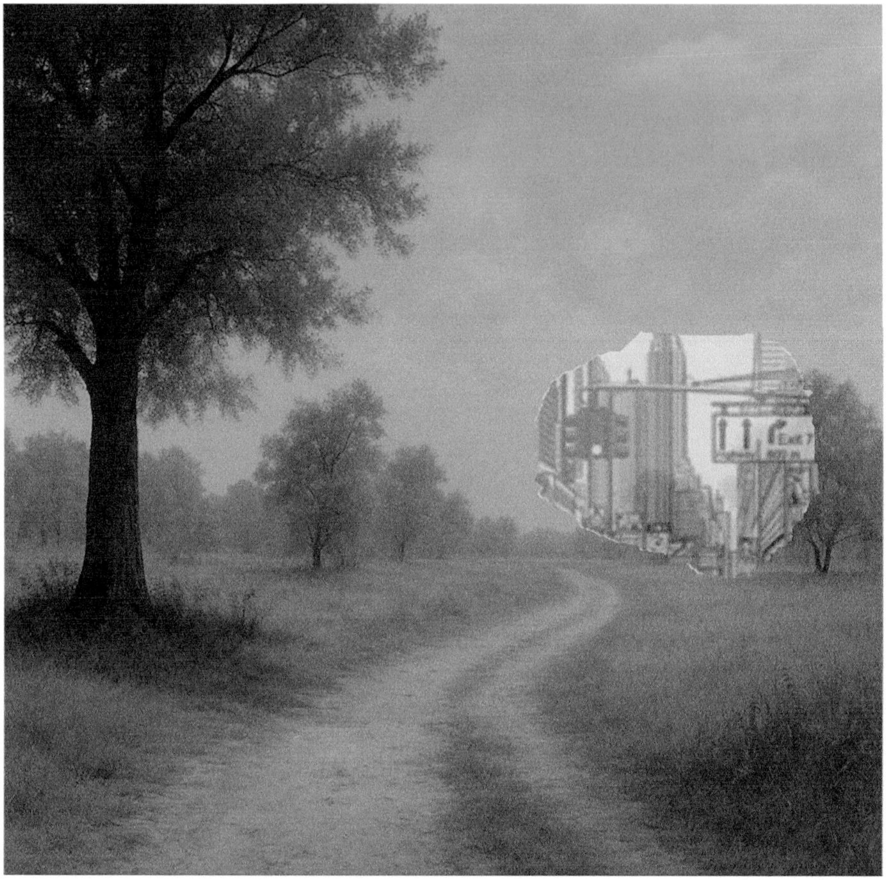

Figure 6.8 Representation of distorted vision seen with palinopsia.

The palinopsic image can be seen by the patient in any location within their visual field.[11] It can remain in the same location as the original image and move as the patient moves their eyes, just as an afterimage would do.[16] It can occupy all or only a portion of the field of vision and is most often limited to the blind field in those patients with homonymous hemianopsia (see Illustrative Case 3).[13] When focal brain lesions have been implicated, they have been predominately right-sided and involve the parietal or occipital lobes, although it is feasible that left hemispheric focal brain lesions may be underrepresented because of the patients' frequently accompanying aphasia.[17–20] Critchley documented right, left, and bilateral intracranial lesions indicating the variability of visual perseveration origin.[10] This phenomenon is very rare and can also occur with stroke, migraine, or as a result of focal seizures.[7, 9, 16] Episodes of palinopsia that result during post-ictal states usually resolve after a few weeks, yet some can persist and these longer acting ones may benefit from a trial of antiepileptic medication.[7, 16, 21]

Illustrative Cases

Illustrative Case 1

A 64-year-old Caucasian female presented to the eye clinic with a complaint of a recent and sudden onset of nonpainful blurred vision in the left eye and a grey defect in the inferior field of vision of the left eye. She felt her right eye was not affected. She had no accompanying headache, temple pain or jaw pain when chewing (jaw claudication). Her medical history was unremarkable, and she was a nonsmoker. Her family history was significant for stroke, all her siblings and both parents had systemic hypertension, and a brother who had fatal valvular heart disease. One of her siblings had a previous episode of nonarteritic anterior ischemic optic neuropathy (NAION) and another had a central retinal artery occlusion.

Her blood pressure was 158/95 right arm sitting position. Her best corrected distance visual acuity was right eye $20/20^{-1}$ and left eye $20/40^{+2}$. On pupil evaluation she had 0.3 log units left relative afferent pupillary defect. Red cap color saturation was equal in both eyes. Her external examination, intraocular pressures and slit-lamp findings were all normal. A dilated fundus evaluation showed a normal right eye except for it having a physiological small cup-to-disc ratio of 0.1. The left optic disc showed superior sectoral edema and a blurred superior disc margin (Figure 6.9a). The optical coherence tomography testing showed a corresponding superior nerve fiber layer swelling in the left eye (Figure 6.9b). A computerized visual field was unremarkable in the right eye and displayed an absolute infranasal altitudinal defect in the left eye (Figure 6.9c). A computerized tomography scan of the head and orbits was negative. A diagnosis of NAION was made since emergent blood testing was negative for arteritic ischemic optic neuropathy (temporal arteritis). NAION is seen in Caucasians older than 50 years who have crowded discs (small cup-to-disc ratio known as a disc-at-risk) and various risk factors such as systemic hypertension, diabetes, obstructive sleep apnea, smoking, etc.

The patient was referred to an internist. A carotid evaluation was negative. She was started on anti-hypertensive medication and an 81mg aspirin. Five weeks later, her disc edema was resolved but the vision and visual field defects remained.

Illustrative Case 2

A 20-year-old male presented to the eye clinic with a complaint of a painless and slow, but progressive, decrease in his distance and near vision in the left eye. He was having difficulty driving and functioning at his construction job. He also had persistent headaches which appeared to be localized behind both his eyes and over the forehead. His medical history was unremarkable. He never had a previous formal eye examination.

His uncorrected visual acuity was right eye 20/30 and left eye 20/400. There was no improvement with pinhole testing. The patient had a trace afferent pupillary defect in the left eye on pupil testing. There were no extraocular muscle

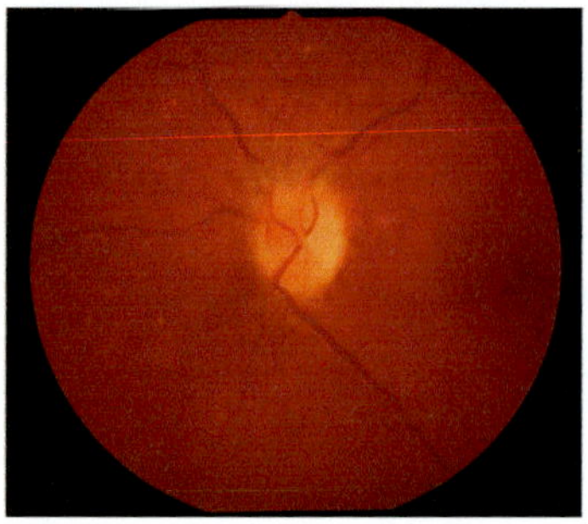

(a)

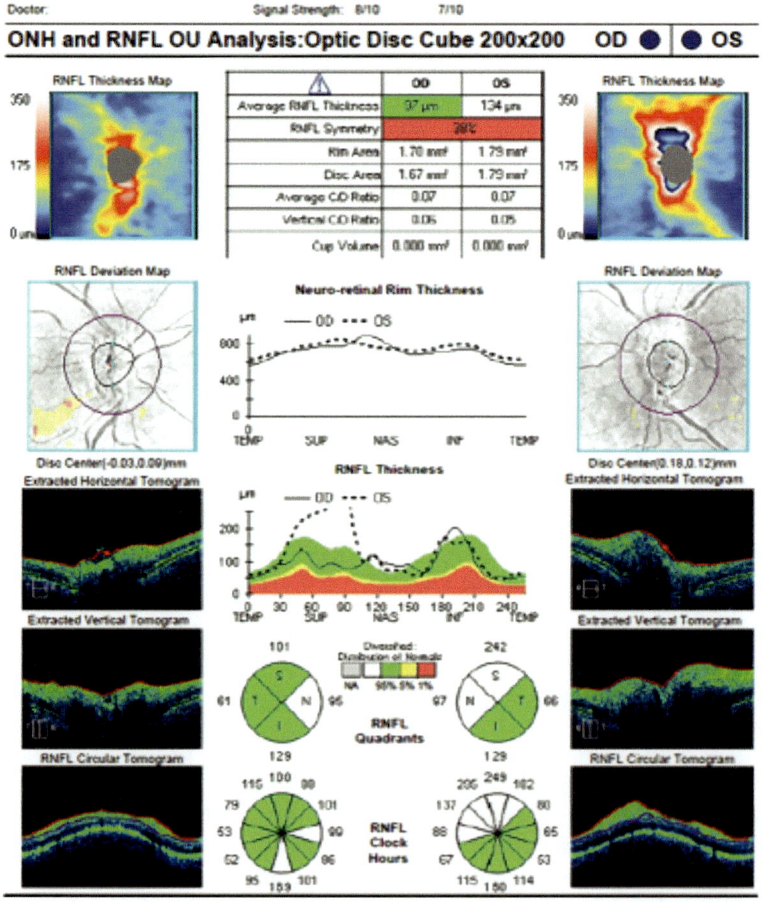

(b)

Figure 6.9 (a) Left optic disc with superior sectoral edema and blurred superior disc margin. (b) Optical coherence tomography showing a corresponding superior nerve fiber layer swelling in the left eye.

(Continued)

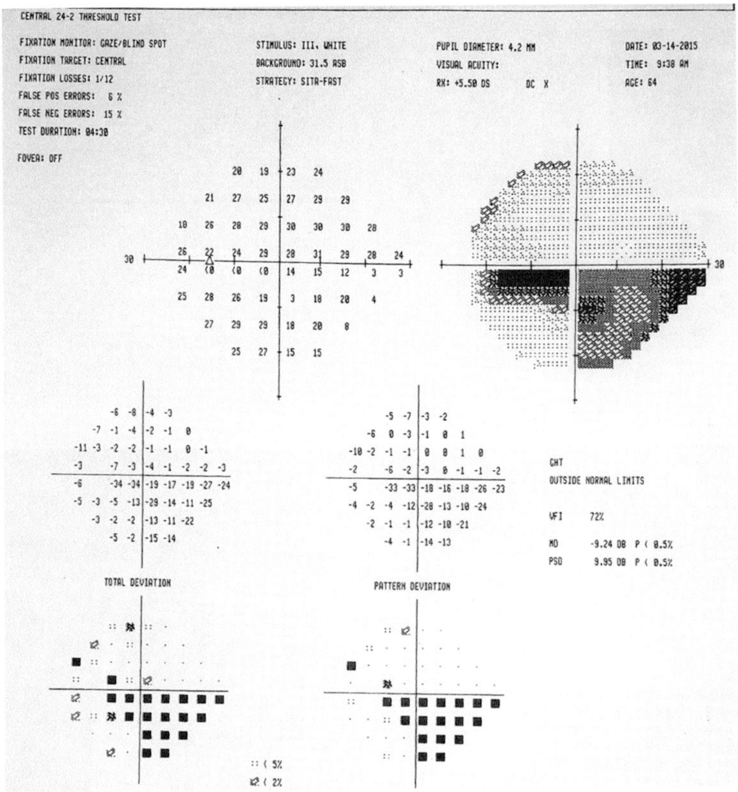

(c)

Figure 6.9 (Continued) (c) Absolute infranasal altitudinal defect in the left eye.

restrictions. Intraocular pressures and slit-lamp examination were normal. The fundus exam was unremarkable in the right eye and the left optic disc showed temporal pallor. A computerized visual field showed bitemporal hemianopsia with extension of the field defect into the nasal quadrant inferiorly in the left eye (Figures 6.10a,b). This type of bitemporal visual defect which respects the vertical meridian localizes the intracranial lesion to the optic chiasm. Neuroimaging revealed an enhancing sellar/suprasellar mass with lateral extension to the left (Figure 6.10c).

Illustrative Case 3

A 34-year-old male was seen as an inpatient at a local hospital. He had suffered a left occipital stroke which was confirmed after admission by magnetic resonance imaging (Figure 6.11a). He felt that his straight-ahead vision was unchanged but that he could no longer see well to his right. Although he was hesitant at first, he said that since his stroke he had been noticing recurrent images of colored circles, dancing fairies, marching men and a man constantly swinging a golf club. He was watching a golf tournament on television while

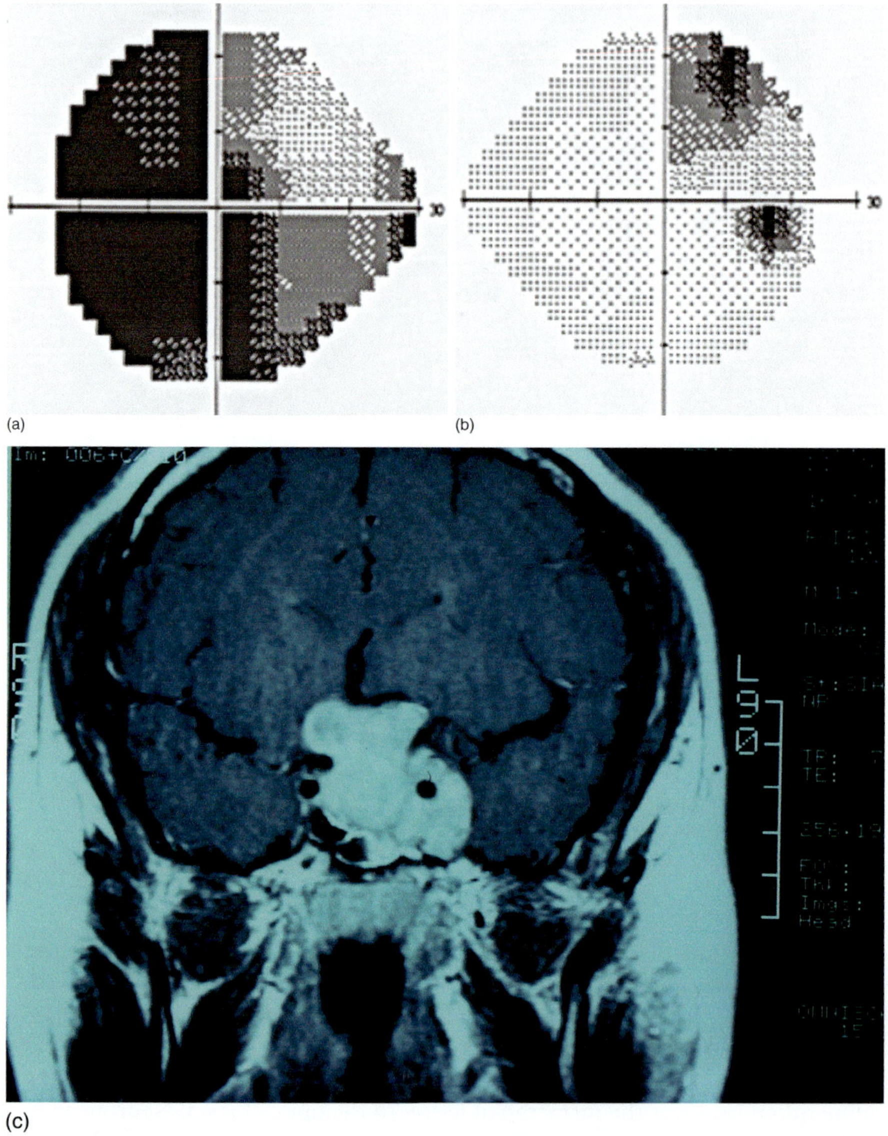

Figure 6.10 (a) Left eye visual field of bitemporal defect with extension into inferior nasal quadrant. (b) Right eye visual field of bitemporal defect. (c) Coronal magnetic resonance imaging of an enhancing sellar-suprasellar mass with lateral extension to the left.

lying in his hospital bed earlier that morning and he recognized the man swinging the golf club continuously as one of the golf tournament contestants. These images appeared exclusively in his right visual field, his blind visual field. (On a subsequent eye examination, he reported seeing recurrent images of one of the chapter authors (LS) approaching with my direct ophthalmoscope, as I had done during my first visit with him when he was an inpatient at the hospital).

His best corrected visual acuity was 20/20 OD and 20/20 OS. The pupil responses were normal. He had no extraocular muscle restrictions and did not exhibit nystagmus. Confrontation visual field testing identified a right homonymous hemianopsia. This was confirmed on a subsequent visit to the eye clinic by automated visual field testing which more specifically showed a right congruous homonymous hemianopsia, denser inferiorly, with macular sparing (Figures 6.11b,c). His intraocular pressures were within normal limits, and a dilated fundus examination was unremarkable.

This patient was describing a classic presentation of palinopsia, especially since his imagery was seen in his blind visual field. The patient was informed that his visual field defect would most likely be permanent. There was no treatment indicated for his visual perseverations since they frequently spontaneously resolve.

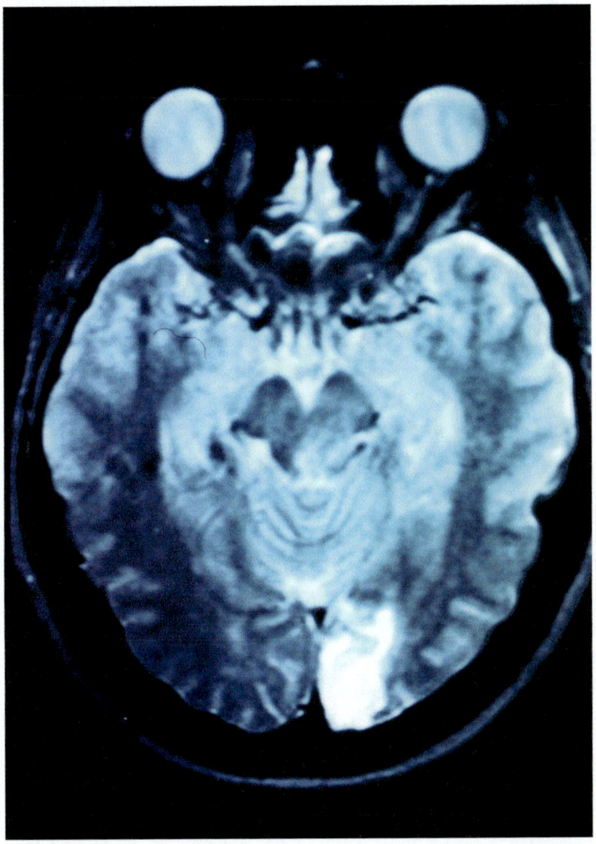

(a)

Figure 6.11 (a) Axial magnetic resonance imaging of left occipital infarction.

(Continued)

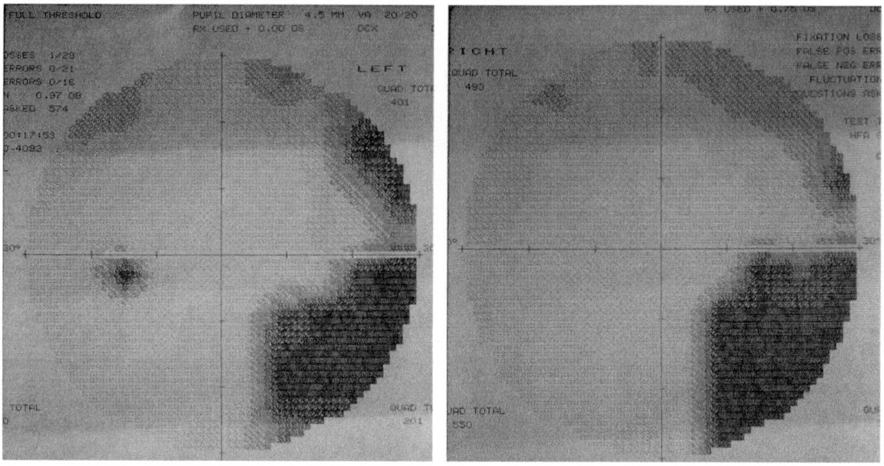

(b) (c)

Figure 6.11 (Continued) (b) Left eye – Right homonymous congruous hemianopsia, denser inferiorly, with macular sparing. (c) Right eye - Right homonymous congruous hemianopsia, denser inferiorly, with macular sparing.

REFERENCES

1. Luckiesh M. *Visual Illusions: Their Causes, Characteristics & Applications*. New York: Dover Publishers; 1965: 1–12.
2. Fraser CL, et al. *Handb Clin Neurol.* 2021. doi: 10.1016/B978-0-12-821377-3.00014-3. PMID: 33832684.
3. Bhatti MT. *2022–2023 BCSC. Vol. 5, Neuro-Ophthalmology*. San Francisco, CA: American Academy of Ophthalmology; 2022.
4. Newman NM. *Neuro-Ophthalmology: A Practical Text.* Norwalk, CT: Appleton & Lange; 1992: 147–50.
5. Martin TJ, et al. *Practical Neuroophthalmology*. New York: McGraw Hill; 2013: 59–84.
6. Cogan DG. Visual hallucinations as release phenomena. *Graefes Arch Klin Exp Ophthalmol.* 1973;188: 139–50.
7. Burde RM, et al. *Clinical Decisions in Neuro-Ophthalmology*, 3rd edn. St. Louis: Mosby; 2002: 114–35.
8. Collerton D, et al. *Neurosci Biobehav Rev.* 2023. doi: 10.1016/j.neubiorev.2023.105208. Epub 2023 May 2. PMID: 37141962.
9. Martin TJ, et al. *Practical Neuroophthalmology*. New York: McGraw Hill; 2013: 319–34.
10. Critchley M. Types of visual perseveration: "Palinopsia" and "illusory spread." *Brain.* 1951;74: 267–99.
11. Rizzo M, et al. Central disorders of visual function. In: Miller NR, Newman NJ, eds. *Walsh & Hoyt's Clinical Neuro-Ophthalmology*, 6th edn. Philadelphia: Lippincott Williams & Wilkins; 2005: 575–645.

12. Jacobs L. Visual allesthesia. *Neurology.* 1980;30: 1059–63.
13. Lessell S, et al. Topical diagnosis: Retrochiasmal visual pathways and higher cortical function. In: Glaser JS, ed. *Neuro-Ophthalmology*, 2nd edn. Philadelphia: J. B. Lippincott Co.; 1990: 213–38.
14. Subramanian P, et al. *Walsh & Hoyt's Clinical Neuro-Ophthalmology: The Essentials*. Philadelphia: Wolters Kluwer Health; 2021. Accessed from: https://research.ebsco.com/linkprocessor/plink?id=ee4ed10d-bab8-32e6-97bb-bd365a9eb64a. Accessed on: 3 February 2025.
15. Kinsbourne M, et al. A study of visual perseveration. *J Neurol Neurosurg Psychiatry.* 1963;26: 468–75.
16. Cummings JL, et al. Palinopsia reconsidered. *Neurology.* 1982;32: 444–7.
17. Bender M, et al. Palinopsia. *Brain.* 1968;91: 321–38.
18. Pane A. *Neuro-Ophthalmology Survival Guide*, 3rd edn. New York, NY Elsevier Limited; 2025: 257–66. E-pub. Accessed on: 3 February 2025.
19. Payne MS. *Hallucinations: Types, Stages and Treatments*. New York: Nova Science Publishers; 2011. Accessed from: https://research.ebsco.com/linkprocessor/plink?id=a1db9e48-3097-388d-b0de-d332a4a57656. Accessed on: 3 February 2025.
20. Shankar Kikkeri N, et al. Migraine with aura. [Updated 2024 Feb 29]. In: *StatPearls* [Internet]. Treasure Island (FL): StatPearls Publishing; 2025 January–. Accessed from: https://www.ncbi.nlm.nih.gov/books/NBK554611/
21. Michel EM, et al. Palinopsia: Cerebral localization with computed tomography. *Neurology.* 1980;30: 887–9.

Chapter 7

HALLUCINATIONS

Leonid Skorin, Jr. and Jesse Britt

Introduction

> "Hallucination, although understood and appreciated as such, by the person under its influence, may, by its frequency and duration, produce so unhappy an effect on the mind as to cause death."[1]
>
> —**Alexandre Brierre de Boismont**

Hallucinations can be defined as subjectively perceived sensory input despite the absence of external stimuli.[2] For visual hallucinations, this presents as seeing something that is physically "not there." In contrast to an illusion, which is considered to be a false interpretation of external reality, visual hallucinations do not disappear with eye closure.[3] Notably, visual hallucinations commonly originate in the retina or visual cortex but may originate from anywhere along the neural portion of the visual pathway. The variety of perceived images can vary drastically depending on what inciting factor or factors are causing an individual to experience visual hallucinations. Furthermore, since visual hallucinations are intrinsically subjective experiences, they are usually inconstant and nebulous, and the individual who perceives them has the difficult task of trying to translate their perceptions into words.[2] From the clinician's perspective, trying to comprehend and analyze the clinical situation of what the patient is experiencing is further confounded by the patient's potential problems with accurate recall, precise description of the visual hallucination, and intentional or unwitting falsification so as not to have the patient labeled as "demented" or "crazy."[2]

Visual hallucinations can be monocular or binocular. Like binocular hemifield illusions, hemifield hallucinations can also be caused by occipitoparietotemporal lesions, transient ischemic attacks, and migraines. Monocular hallucinations are always due to abnormalities of the optic nerve or the photoreceptors.[3] Images that are seen can be as simple as dots, spots, streaks or lines, or they can be as complex as faces, animals, cars, or landscapes. Thus, visual hallucinations are typically separated into two broad categories: unformed (also known as simple or elementary) and formed (also known as complex).

DOI: 10.1201/9781003633365-7

Unformed Hallucinations

i. Phosphenes

Phosphenes, the false perception of light, is a photopsia that typically presents as colored or colorless bright lights such as points, flashes of light, stars, sparks, streaks, or even resembling lightning (Moore's lightning streaks, which result from traction of the vitreous on the peripheral retina) (Figure 7.1).[4] These phenomena occur in the setting of photoreceptor deformation. This can be seen with retinal tear and/or retinal detachment, vitreous detachment, intraocular tumor, or induced by eye movement. Some phosphenes can be induced by sound and are referred to as auditory-visual synesthetic phenomena.[5,6] Incidences of sound-induced, eye

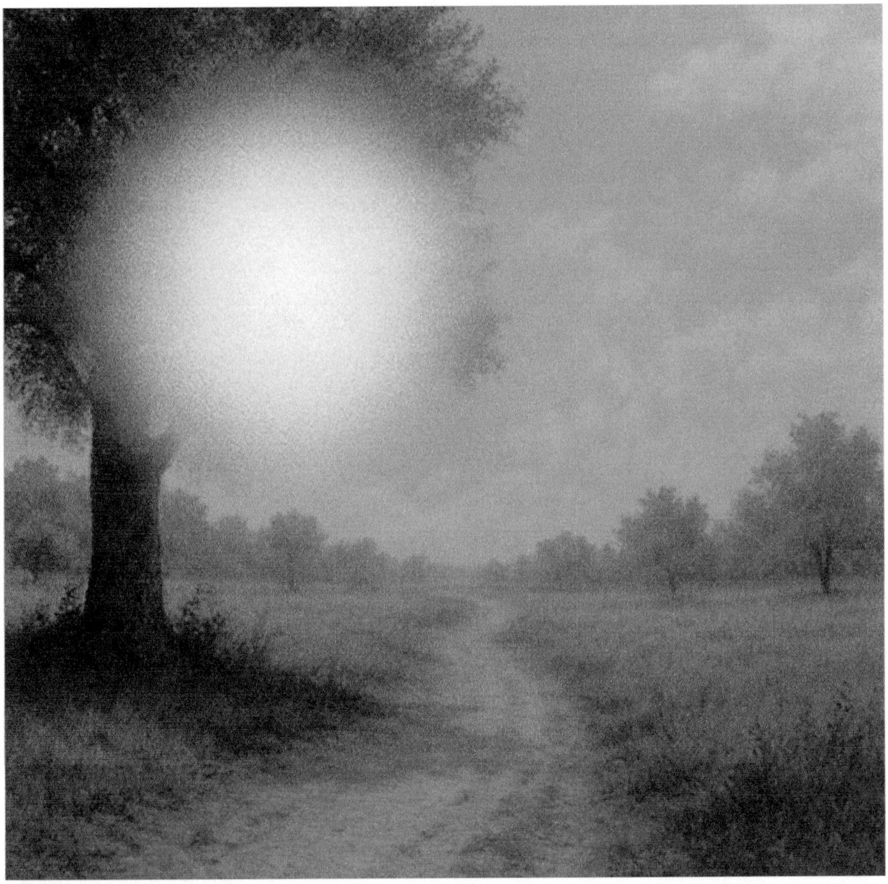

Figure 7.1 Representation of a phosphene, an unformed visual hallucination commonly seen in classic migraine.

movement-induced or even spontaneous phosphenes in the presence of optic neuropathy that most probably resulted from a demyelinating event such as optic neuritis have been readily noted.[7] Flickering lights or visual "snow" (silvery scintillations) is another form of photopsia that patients may describe. This can be from inflammation such as multiple evanescent white dot syndrome, retinal ischemia from either artery or venous occlusion, optic neuropathy either from an ischemic or a demyelinating event such as optic neuritis, retinal degeneration such as retinitis pigmentosa, and sometimes migraine.[8–11] In those cases where there is no obvious etiology, the term visual snow syndrome (VSS) can be used. VSS is persistent in many of these patients and occurs regardless of the surrounding lighting conditions. It fits the definition of a visual hallucination since it continues to be present even when the eyes are closed. It has been described as looking through static as seen in an untuned television or seeing flickering white or transparent dots or spots in a snow globe after it has been shaken, but where the "snow" never settles to the bottom of the snow globe (Figure 7.2). A recent study

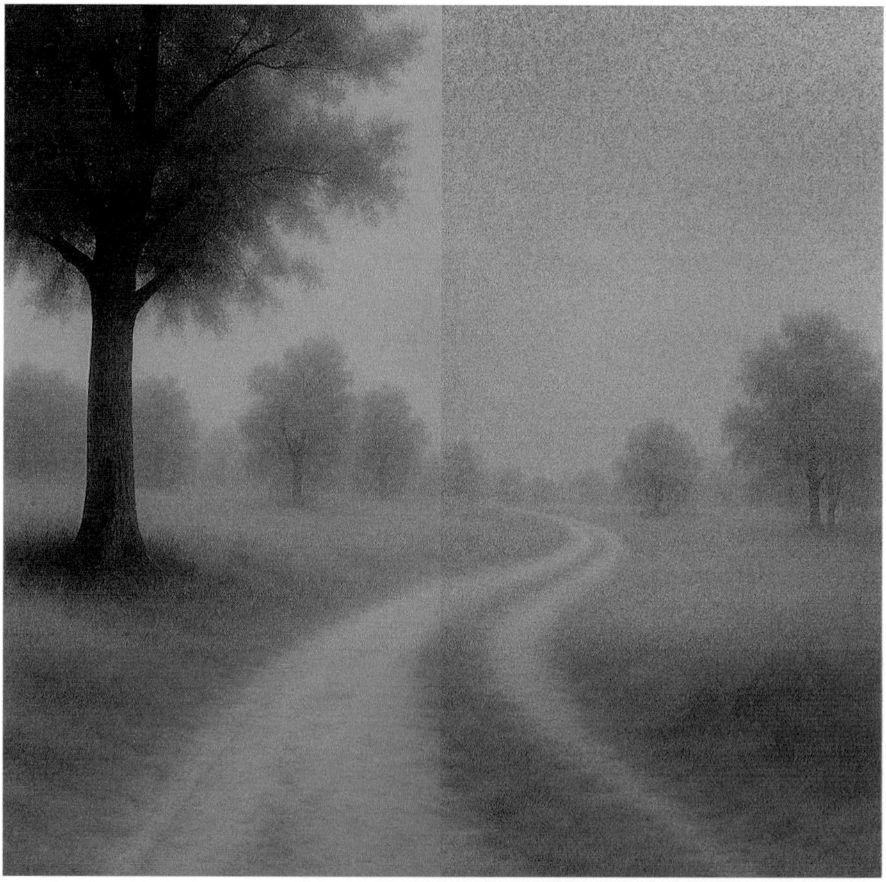

Figure 7.2 Visual snow syndrome. Image on the left shows scene as it truly is and image on the right is what a patient with visual snow syndrome would see.

has estimated that up to 2% of the general population in the United Kingdom have VSS.[12] VSS is considered to be chronic in nature and may be accompanied with migraines, anxiety, depression, and tinnitus.[12–14]

ii. Chromatopsia (Chromopia, Chromopsia, Chromopsy)

Chromatopsia is the abnormal perception of color vision where an individual sees things in a single hue or tinged with that color. The various chromatopsias are designated according to the color that is seen: xanthopsia, brunescence, erythropsia (also known as erythropia), cyanopsia (also known as cyanopia), chloropsia (also known as chloropia), and ianthinopsia (also known as ianthopsia or ianothinopsia).

- Xanthopsia, or yellow vision, is the most common change seen in color vision.[15] Xanthopsia may occur in patients who use digoxin or digitoxin. It occurs in about 80% of patients who have digoxin intoxication (the experience of nausea, vomiting, abdominal discomfort, and cardiac arrhythmias), but can also be detected in individuals who are at therapeutic drug levels.[16] The Farnsworth–Munsell 100-hue test has been shown to be particularly sensitive for detecting digitalis-induced color vision deficiencies.[16] In addition to xanthopsia, visual symptoms in digitalis intoxication may include a patient experiencing a blue tinge in their vision with or without colored halos, colored spots surrounded by coronas, snowy, hazy, or blurred vision, dimming of vision, flickering or flashes of light, and increased glare sensitivity.[17]
- A common complaint heard in patients with cataracts is that everything, but especially white carpets, clothing, counter tops, etc., have a dingy yellow brownish tint. This is known as brunescence and although many cataract patients complain of this before having successful cataract surgery, many will not realize the true extent of this brunescent color aberration until after their successful cataract surgery (see Illustrative Case).[3]
- Erythropsia (or red-tinted vision) is nearly always associated with hemorrhages in the anterior chamber, vitreous, or retina of the eye.[18] Erythropsia can occur in patients who use atropine, ergotamine, and various sulfa drugs.[16] Erythropsias may also affect aphakes and pseudophakes after exposure to bright sun or snow.[19] Without evidence of ocular abnormality, erythropsia is likely psychogenic.[3]
- Cyanopsia is blue-tinted vision which can occur with the systemic use of amphetamines, chloroquine, digitalis, nalidixic acid, ethionamide, oral contraceptives, and medications that are used to treat erectile dysfunction such as phosphodiesterase-5 inhibitors.[16] Patients who undergo cataract surgery and intraocular lens implantation may initially, after the surgery, report seeing a blue tint on and around objects. The natural crystalline lens with a cataract absorbs the blue light wavelength. After the cataract surgery, the intraocular lens implant lets the full spectrum of light into the eye, and the patient now sees the blue light (the blue light wavelength was previously blocked by the cataract) as an exaggerated perception (see Illustrative Case).[20]

- Chloropsia (green-tinted vision) and ianthinopsia (violet-tinted or purple vision) are exceedingly rare.[21] Chloropsia and ianthinopsia have been seen with digitalis toxicity.[16]
- Cerebral achromatopsia (also known as central achromatopsia) is a form of acquired color blindness that is caused by damage to the bilateral visual cortex and its connections and needs to be distinguished from the hereditary autosomal recessive genetic condition that causes total color blindness from birth.[22] Cerebral achromatopsia is most frequently caused by conditions acquired later in life such as trauma, including any resulting concussion, tumor, or hemorrhage.[23] One interesting and detailed case is presented by neurologist and author Oliver Sacks. This involved an artist who specialized in doing colorful paintings and who unfortunately acquired color blindness after the artist had been involved in an automobile accident in which he sustained a concussion, transient amnesia, and temporary alexia in addition to his permanent total color vision deficit.[24] In cases of unilateral occipital damage, a hemiachromatopsia may result where there is a loss of color vision in the contralateral half of the visual field.[25] Color sorting or matching tests, such as the Farnsworth–Munsell 100-Hue Test and the Farnsworth D-15, provide the clinician the best evidence of this type of impaired color perception in bilateral cases while patients with hemiachromatopsia often score normally on these tests.[25]

iii. Fortification Spectrum (Teichopsia)

Patients who experience migraines may see unformed hallucinations. Migraine without aura (common migraine) is characterized by onset of hemicranial or generalized headache without any focal neurologic symptoms such as visual hallucinations occurring prior to the headache or accompanying the head pain. In patients who have migraine with aura (classic migraine), the visual phenomenon usually precedes or accompanies the headache, whereas in the acephalgic migraine or migraine equivalent, the visual phenomenon occurs without the patient developing a headache afterwards.[25] Patients with any of these migraine variants may experience a premonitory phase and a resolution phase which present as hyperactivity, hypoactivity, depression, food cravings, or repetitive yawning.[25] Although these migraineurs may see phosphenes such as spots, wavy lines, a shimmering, like heat waves over a road on a hot day, visual distortion like water running down a windowpane or even arborizations (dendropsies), the teichopsia or fortification spectrum is the classic pattern described by many.[25] It takes the shape of an arc of light (C-shaped, sickle-shaped or bean-shaped) with formations of dazzling zigzag lines which resemble the battlements of a castle or fortified walls of a medieval fortress, hence the name, fortification spectrum.[18, 26] The "spectrum" part of the term comes from the ephemeral nature of this visual hallucination and it's spectral or ghostly quality.[26] The name teichopsia bares its roots from the Greek word *teichos*, meaning "city wall."[26] These zigzag lines begin near central vision and expand (buildup or march) toward the periphery with increasing speed over the next 20–30 minutes in an oscillating or scintillating fashion.[25, 27] This "scintillating scotoma" is a blind region surrounded by a margin of luminous sparkling lights which occurs bilaterally, but involving only one homonymous hemifield, pointing to its origin in the visual cortex (Figure 7.3).[25, 28] In their wake they leave scotomatous defects in the field of vision while the throbbing or pounding head pain begins as the visual hallucination resolves.[18] In some cases, migraine-related unformed visual hallucinations may be more elaborate than simply flashing lights and may include lines, webs, lattice formations, tunneling imagery, spirals, pinwheels, and kaleidoscopic forms.[29] In rare cases, fortification spectra can arise from pathological intracranial etiologies, such as vertebrobasilar insufficiency, occipital lobe arteriovenous malformations, or meningiomas.[18] Unlike in migraineurs, these hallucinations will be accompanied by bruits, persistent hemianopsias, seizures, and headaches experienced consistently on

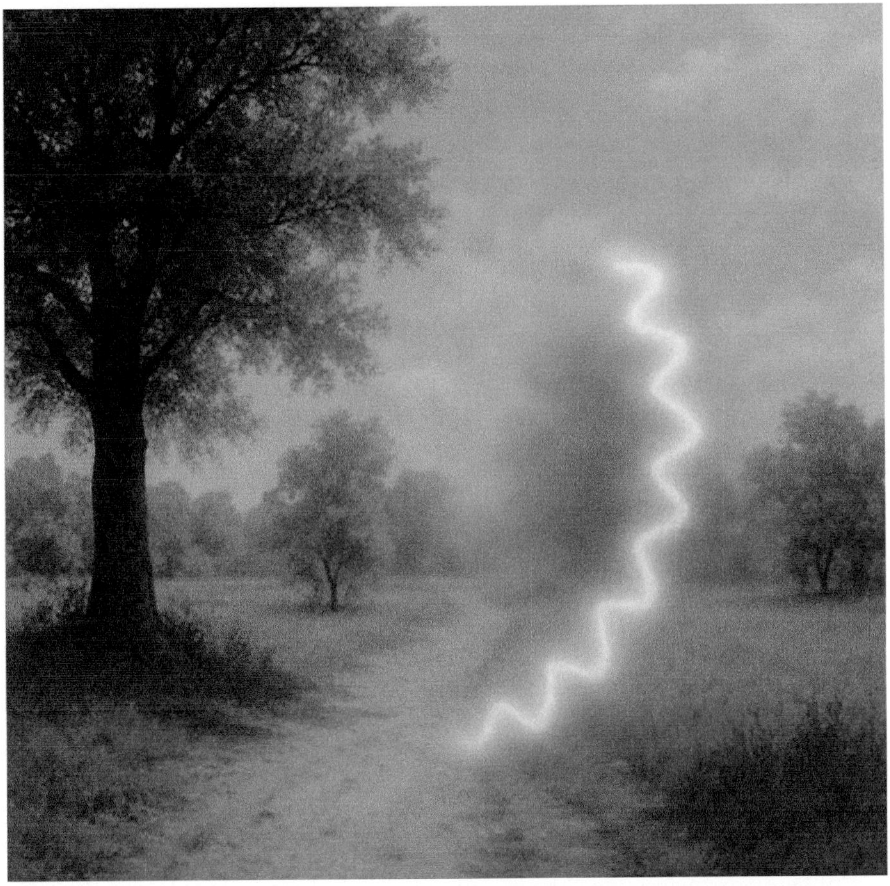

Figure 7.3 Representation of scintillating scotoma, an unformed visual hallucination commonly seen in classic migraine.

one side of the head.[18] Another important clinical difference is that these headaches will not respond to any of the usual medication.[15] Patients who exhibit these serious signs and symptoms warrant a neurologic evaluation, including neuroimaging of the brain.

Formed Hallucinations

Unlike simpler unformed hallucinations, formed hallucinations are more complex. These types of visual anomalies typically involve processes such as metamorphopsia, micropsia, macropsia, teleopsia, pelopsia, microsomatognosia, macrosomatognosia, mosaic vision, and Alice in Wonderland syndrome. Etiologies of these abnormalities include, but are not limited to refractive problems, retinal deformation, maculopathy, cerebral lesions, and migraine.

i. **Metamorphopsia**

Metamorphopsia is the distortion of an image in shape, size, location, or color. For example, instead of seeing the straight lines of structures such as door frames or telephone poles or patterns such as straight horizontal lines on lined paper and columns of print in newspapers or books, the patient sees curvilinear distortion. It can be from retinal causes (i.e. retinal metamorphopsia) or cerebral causes (i.e. cerebral metamorphopsia). Retinal metamorphopsias tend to occur from disruption of the cones, which are photoreceptors located in the macula of the retina. Cones can be displaced by degeneration, scarring, inflammation, edema, hemorrhage, vitreous traction, etc. Among examples of ocular diseases that can affect the macula and cause retinal metamorphopsia are age-related macular degeneration, central serous chorioretinopathy, pseudophakic cystoid macular edema, diabetic maculopathy, and epiretinal membrane, which is also known as macular pucker. Patients with retinal metamorphopsia will only notice distortion in their central vision. Unfortunately, since our most precise and acute vision is formed from these photoreceptors in the macula, these patients will usually also notice a significant worsening of their visual acuity. Their peripheral vision remains unaffected and without any metamorphopsia. Retinal metamorphopsia can be easily evaluated by the clinician with the use of the Amsler grid that allows the detection and localization of distortion in the central visual field (Figure 7.4).[30] Since the Amsler grid is a hand-held card, it also allows the patient to self-monitor the central visual field for the development of visual symptoms or their changes.[30] Cones that get displaced farther apart tend to create the illusion of objects appearing smaller than they are (retinal micropsia), whereas cones that get pushed closer together generate a perceived image that is larger than reality (retinal macropsia). Retinal micropsia is usually associated with eye diseases that cause macular edema and these patients also often have retinal metamorphopsia and decreased visual acuity. Retinal macropsia occurs much less frequently than retinal micropsia and is usually a result of late scarring seen in chronic untreated macular edema.[25] In the absence of identifiable maculopathy after an eye examination, the underlying etiology is likely psychogenic or intracranial in nature.

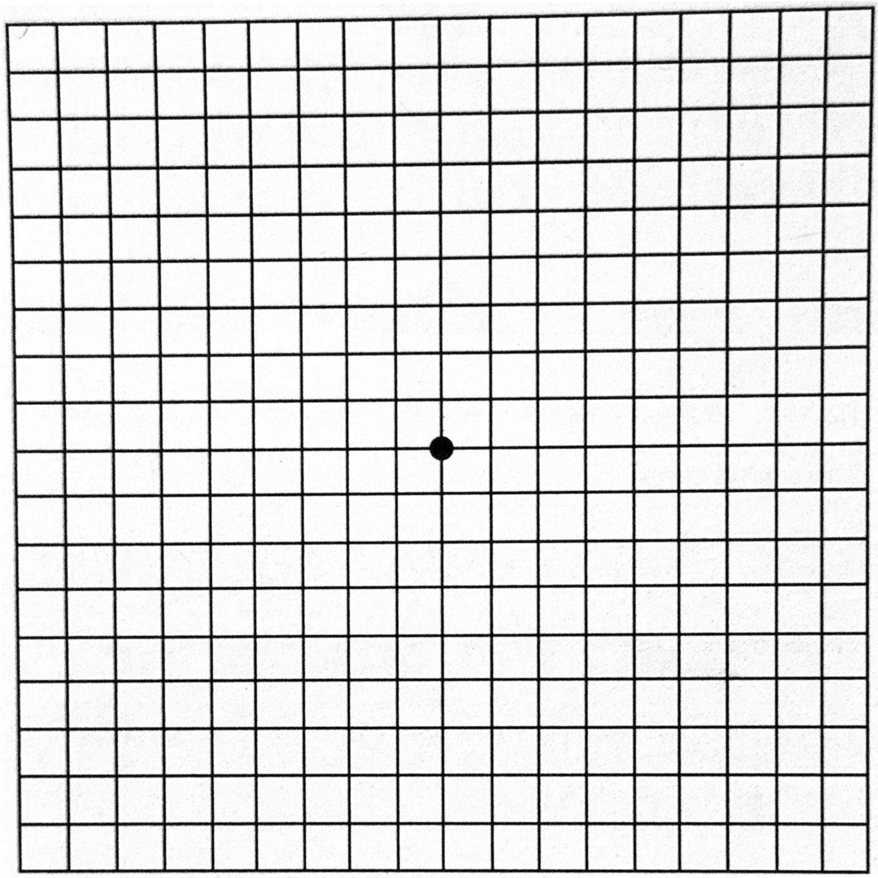

Figure 7.4 Amsler grid, a handheld card that allows the detection and localization of distortion in the central visual field.

Cerebral metamorphopsia tends to produce more drastic visual changes, resulting in grossly distorted perception of viewed objects involving the complete field and not just the central field as seen in retinal metamorphopsia. It can be intermittent or persistent, depending on the underlying cause. Intracranially oriented etiologies, such as seizures, tumors, arteriovenous malformations and infarction, have all been implicated in causing cerebral metamorphopsia.[25] It is often seen with a concomitant palinopsia. An unusual form of cerebral metamorphopsia is the inversion illusion, also known as room-tilt illusion or upside-down vision.[31] These patients develop a sudden and transient 180-degree rotation of the visual image in the coronal plane.[31] Underlying causes for this phenomenon include some sort of hypoperfusion or complete infarct of the intracranial posterior circulation including the vestibular system, but has also occurred from migraine, focal seizures, and concussion (Figures 7.5a,b).[31]

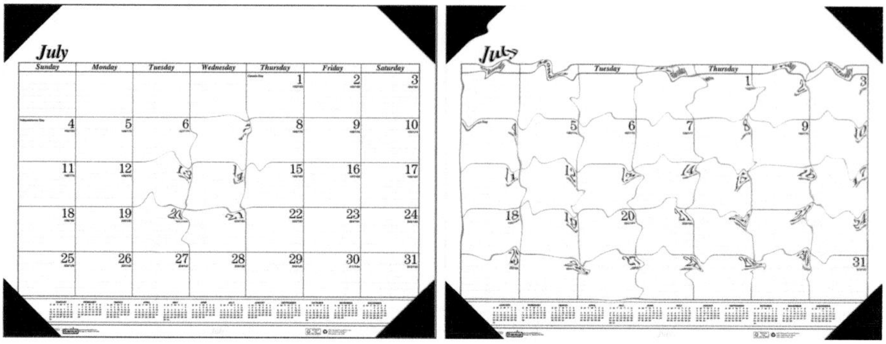

(a) (b)

Figure 7.5 (a) Distorted vision involving only the central visual field as seen with retinal/macular metamorphopsia. (b) Distorted vision involving the whole visual field as seen with cerebral metamorphopsia.

ii. Alice in Wonderland Syndrome

Alice in Wonderland syndrome is a dysmetropsia, which is a disorder of image size and/or location that occurs in both eyes but has a visual cortex origin. Individuals who experience complex migraine-related visual hallucinations almost always learn not to mistake these perceptual disturbances for reality.[29] Alice in Wonderland syndrome is named after the children's novel, *Alice's Adventures in Wonderland* written by the English author Charles Lutwidge Dodgson (Lewis Carroll), who relived the memories of his own auras and classic migraine attacks when he created the characters of this book.[32] Lewis Carroll's descriptions of the various size and location perceptual disturbances, which occur to the various characters within this book, appear as extraordinarily graphic and accurate representations of the complex formed visual hallucinations seen occasionally in migraineurs during the aura stage of the headache.[32]

A wide array of formed visual hallucinations can be seen in Alice in Wonderland syndrome. Some, such as cerebral metamorphopsia, micropsia, macropsia, and the inversion illusion, have already been addressed in the previous section. Mention should be made about Lilliputianism, where an individual perceives people around them as appearing smaller than they really are. This is named after the miniature inhabitants of the island of Lilliput from the novel *Gulliver's Travels* written by Jonathan Swift. Therefore, these miniaturizations can be referred to as either Lilliputian images or Gulliverian hallucinations. The neurologist and author Oliver Sacks wonders if these Lilliputian visual hallucinations, which he regards as not uncommon, potentially give rise to stories of elves, dwarfs, imps, leprechauns, Hawaiian *menehune* and fairies in our folklore, art, and even religion.[33] Different forms of this disturbance can affect self-perception, where the individual has difficulty correctly perceiving the size and feel of either their whole body or only specific body parts. This may include the

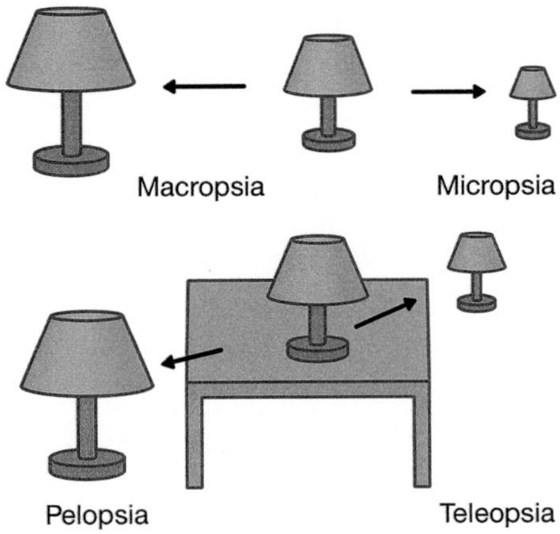

Figure 7.6 Depiction of various types of Alice in Wonderland syndrome effects. Macropsia (lamp shade image seen larger than it really is); Micropsia (lamp shade image seen smaller than it really is); Pelopsia (lamp shade image displaced closer than it really is); Teleopsia (lamp shade image is displaced further than it really is).

feeling that one is shorter or taller or perceptions of a body part as anomalously smaller than it is (microsomatognosia) or conversely perceiving a body part as anomalously larger than it is (macrosomatognosia).[34] Patients have described feeling as if a part of the body, such as the neck, the ear, or the hip, "balloons out," or the head feels as if it were enlarged and floating toward the ceiling.[34, 35] If there is an accompanying field defect such as a scotoma, these distorted body parts may be superimposed within the scotoma.[29] Teleopsia is the name given to the condition when objects are perceived as farther away, while pelopsia is when objects are perceived as being closer than they really are (Figure 7.6).

Other more rare visual hallucinations in migraine that are considered as being complex or present as visual illusions include cerebral polyopia (seeing multiple identical copies of a single image), visual perseveration (the reoccurrence of previously seen images), visual allesthesia (seeing the image of an object that was previously viewed as being displaced from one homonymous hemifield into the contralateral hemifield), autokinesis (illusory movement of self), cinematographic vision (perceiving scenes as rapidly flickering series of "stills" like in a slide show), corona phenomenon (an extra contour around objects), facial metamorphopsia (alteration of the affective assessment of the extracorporeal environment, rendering it either beautiful, ugly or frightening), illusory vertical splitting, tilted vision, other forms of illusory rotation, vision loss, and mosaic vision.[25, 29] Mosaic vision is the fracturing into pieces of an image into irregular, crystalline, polygonal facets that are joined together as in a "mosaic" (Figure 7.7).[36]

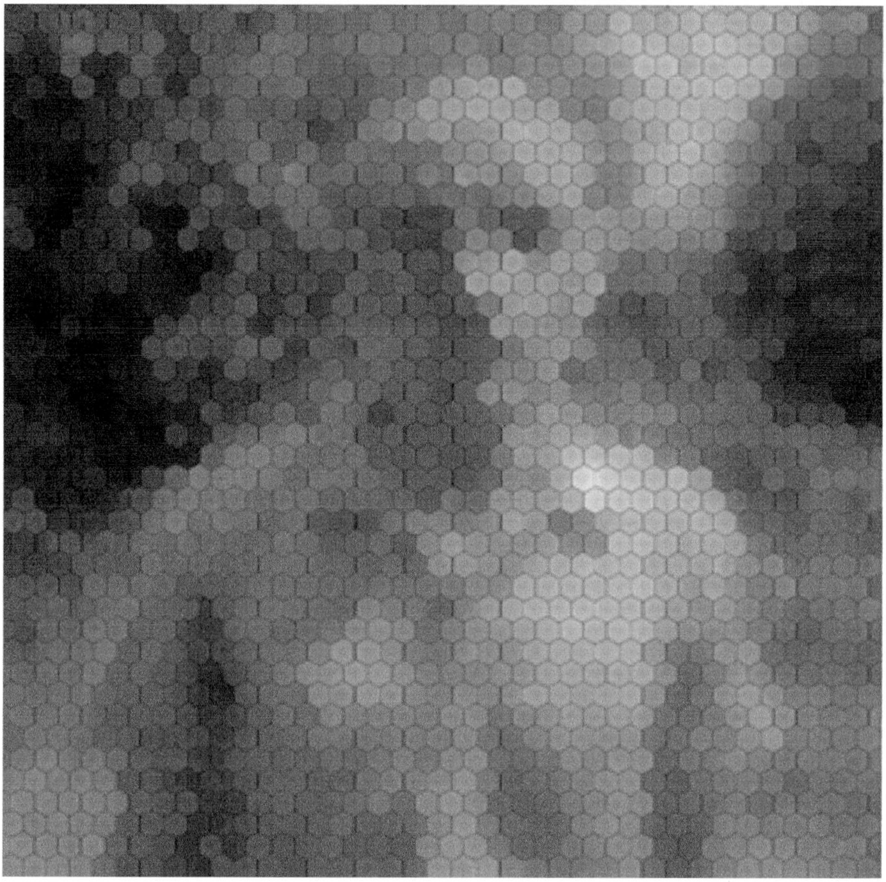

Figure 7.7 Representation of mosaic vision.

Illustrative Case

A 67-year-old female complained of painless worsening of her vision in both eyes. This vision loss gradually progressed over about one year to the point that she was having difficulty seeing driving safely. She also stated that all her colors were muted and everything looked dingy. Her optometrist could no longer strengthen her glasses prescription to improve her vision in either eye, and had therefore referred her for cataract surgery. The patient's ocular history included high myopia, vitreous floaters and dry eye. She was using various over-the-counter dry eye drops on an "as needed" basis for her dry eye symptoms. Her medical history included mild hypertension and dyslipidemia, both of which were well controlled with medication.

Her best-corrected visual acuity was 20/80 right eye and 20/200 left eye. Her pupil evaluation, extraocular motility, intraocular pressures, and confrontation visual fields were normal. On slit-lamp examination the patient was found to have 2+–3+ nuclear sclerotic, 1+ cortical and 2+ posterior subcapsular cataracts in both eyes. The dilated fundus examination found vitreous syneresis with vitreous floaters, myopic-appearing optic discs but no retinal pathology in either eye. The patient was scheduled for cataract surgery, starting with her worse-seeing left eye.

After successful left eye cataract surgery with intraocular lens implantation, the patient's visual acuity was improved to 20/40 uncorrected, but for the first week postoperatively she noted that everything she saw out of that eye was tinted blue. The patient was reassured that this would resolve as the eye healed. On her one-week postoperative visit, her vision in the left eye could be corrected to 20/20 and she no longer had her blue-tinted vision. She also noted that she could now see true blues and greens more vividly and the dingy brownish yellow haze was no longer present when she looked only through the left eye. These visual acuity and color changes were significantly noticeable for her when she compared her vision between her surgically corrected left eye and the eye which still had a cataract. Interestingly, after her second eye cataract surgery, the patient experienced cyanopsia again, this time in the right eye for one-week postoperatively. After this period, the cyanopsia and original brunescence had been resolved.

REFERENCES

1. de Boismont AB. *Hallucinations: Or, The Rational History of Apparitions, Visions, Dreams, Ecstasy, Magnetism, and Somnambulism*. Philadelphia: Lindsay and Blakiston; 1853: 40–75. Special edition from *The Classics of Psychiatry & Behavioral Sciences Library*. New York: Gryphon Editions; 1995.
2. Bliss EL, et al. Visual hallucinations. In: West LJ, ed. *Hallucinations*. New York: Grune & Stratton; 1962: 92–107.
3. Burde RM, et al. *Clinical Decisions in Neuro-Ophthalmology*, 3rd edn. St. Louis: Mosby; 2002: 114–35.
4. Menon GJ, et al. Complex visual hallucinations in the visually impaired: The Charles Bonnet syndrome. *Surv Ophthalmol*. 2003;48(1): 58–72.
5. Jacobs L, et al. Auditory-visual synesthesia: Sound-induced photisms. *Arch Neurol*. 1981;38: 211–16.
6. Page NGR, et al. Auditory evoked phosphenes in optic nerve disease. *J Neurol Neurosurg Psychiatry*. 1982;45: 7–12.
7. Pardo G. Multiple sclerosis and optic neuritis. *Focal Points: Clinical Modules for Ophthalmologists. Am Acad Ophthalmol*. 2003;21(12): 1–13.
8. Jampol LM, et al. Multiple evanescent white dot syndrome. *I. Clinical findings. Arch Ophthalmol*. 1984;102: 671–4.
9. Furlan AJ, et al. Unilateral visual loss in bright light: An unusual symptom of carotid artery occlusive disease. *Arch Neurol*. 1979;36: 675–6.
10. Abel A, et al. Critical review: Typical and atypical optic neuritis. *Surv Ophthalmol*. 2019;64(6): 770–9.

11. Brown GC, et al. Photopsias: A key diagnosis. *Ophthalmology*. 2015;122(10): 2084–94.
12. Kondziella D, et al. Prevalence of visual snow syndrome in the UK. *Eur J Neurol*. 2020;27: 764–72.
13. Puledda F, et al. Visual snow syndrome: A clinical and phenotypical description of 1,100 cases. *Neurology*. 2020;94(6): e564–e574.
14. van Dongen RM, et al. Treatment effects and comorbid diseases in 58 patients with visual snow. *Neurology*. 2019;93: e398–e403.
15. Lessell S. Visual hallucinations and related phenomena. *Neur Neurosurg*. 1979;2: 48–53.
16. Prokopich CL, et al. Ocular adverse drug reactions to systemic medications. In: Bartlett JD, Jaanus SD, eds. *Clinical Ocular Pharmacology*, 5th edn. St. Louis: Butterworth Heinemann Elsevier; 2008: 701–59.
17. Weleber RG, et al. Digoxin retinal toxicity: Clinical and electrophysiological evaluation of a cone dysfunction syndrome. *Arch Ophthalmol*. 1981;99: 1568–72.
18. Skorin L. Visual hallucinations: Perception as deception. *Rev Optom*. 1993;130(12): 30–2.
19. Sternberg P, et al. Blizzard of '83 erythropsia [Letter]. *N Engl J Med*. 1983;308: 1482–3.
20. Skorin L. Disorder has patients "seeing things". *Rev Optom*. 2005;142(10): 49–55.
21. Pinckers A, et al. Chromatopsia. *Doc Ophthalmologica*. 1989;72: 385–90.
22. Zeki S. A century of cerebral achromatopsia. *Brain*. 1990;113: 1721–77.
23. Bouvier SE, et al. Behavioral deficits and cortical damage loci in cerebral achromatopsia. *Neuropsychologia*. 2006;16(2): 183–91.
24. Sacks O. *An Anthropologist on Mars: Seven Paradoxical Tales*. New York: Vintage Books; 1995: 3–41.
25. Rizzo M, et al. Central disorders of visual function. In: Miller NR, Newman NJ, eds. *Walsh & Hoyt's Clinical Neuro-Ophthalmology*, 6th edn. Philadelphia: Lippincott Williams & Wilkins; 2005: 575–645.
26. Plant GT. The fortification spectra of migraine. *Br Med J*. 1986;293: 1613–7.
27. Lessell S, et al. Topical diagnosis: Retrochiasmal visual pathways and higher cortical function. In: Glaser JS, ed. *Neuro-Ophthalmology*, 2nd edn. Philadelphia: J. B. Lippincott Co.; 1990: 213–38.
28. Adams RD, et al. *Principles of Neurology*, 5th edn. New York: McGraw-Hill; 1993: 148–70.
29. Onofrj M, et al. The clinical associations of visual hallucinations. In: Collerton D, Mosimann UP, Perry E, eds. *The Neuroscience of Visual Hallucinations*. Oxford: Wiley Blackwell; 2015: 91–117.
30. Rihani HT, et al. Age-related macular degeneration. In: Onofrey BE, Skorin L, Holdeman NR, eds. *Ocular Therapeutics Handbook: A Clinical Manual*, 4th edn. Philadelphia: Wolters Kluwer; 2020: 514–9.

31. Mullen C, et al. Turning the world upside down: Reversal-of-vision metamorphopsia in a patient with syncope. *BMJ Case Rep.* 2023;16(12): e255453. doi: 10.1136/bcr-2023-255453.
32. Cady RK, et al. Introduction. In: Cady RK, Fox AW, eds. *Treating the Headache Patient.* New York: Marcel Dekker; 1995: 1–14.
33. Sacks O. *Hallucinations.* New York: Alfred A. Knopf; 2012: xii, 102.
34. Davidoff RA. *Migraine: Manifestations, Pathogenesis, and Management.* Philadelphia: F. A. Davis Co.; 1995: 44–76.
35. Lippman CW. Certain hallucinations peculiar to migraine. *J Nerv Ment Dis.* 1952;116: 346–51.
36. Hadjikhani N, et al. *Vision (Basel).* 2021. doi: 10.3390/vision5020020. PMID: 33924855; PMCID: PMC8167726.

Chapter 8

CHARLES BONNET SYNDROME

Gary M. Cusick and Leonid Skorin, Jr.

Introduction

> "In general, people are afraid to acknowledge hallucinations because they immediately see them as a sign of something awful happening to the brain, whereas in most cases they're not.[1]"
>
> —Oliver Sacks

Charles Bonnet and His Grandfather, Charles Lullin

The Swiss naturalist Charles Bonnet (1720–1793) (Figure 8.1) was a polymath who did research and published studies in the areas of entomology, botany, psychology, philosophy (metaphysics), and the law despite having become deaf at age seven.[2–5] His work in entomology and his theory of parthenogenesis earned him admittance to the French Academy of Science in 1740 and to the London Royal Society in London in 1743.[6] He proposed a theory of evolution 100 years before the publication of Darwin's *On the Origin of Species*.[7]

In 1760 he published a book, *Essai Analytique sur les Facultés de L'âme—Analytical Essay on the Powers of the Soul*, in which he described visual hallucinations that his cognitively intact 89-year-old grandfather, Charles Lullin experienced after significant sight loss.[8] Lullin was a retired magistrate whose vision deteriorated after unsuccessful cataract surgery in both eyes.[9] He initially saw simple visual hallucinations resembling a blue handkerchief with a small yellow circle in each corner.[10] Six months later, he started seeing complex images such as people, including men wearing cloaks and hats and women fully adorned with colorful ribbons and jewelry, and occasionally wearing small boxes on their exquisitely coifed heads.[9, 10] He also saw birds, carriages, buildings and other structures such as scaffolding that changed in shape, size (becoming gigantic or miniaturized) and place.[9, 10] In addition, Lullin experienced autoscopia, where he saw an image of himself.[9] Bonnet recorded that his grandfather was completely mentally intact and realized that what he saw was not real but simply visual hallucinations.[9–11]

Bonnet contracted an "eye ailment" and developed cataracts, making it impossible for him to use a microscope for his entomological studies; eventually, he was unable to either read or write.[9] Later in his life, Bonnet developed what became known in 1936 as Charles Bonnet Syndrome (CBS) himself after experiencing

DOI: 10.1201/9781003633365-8

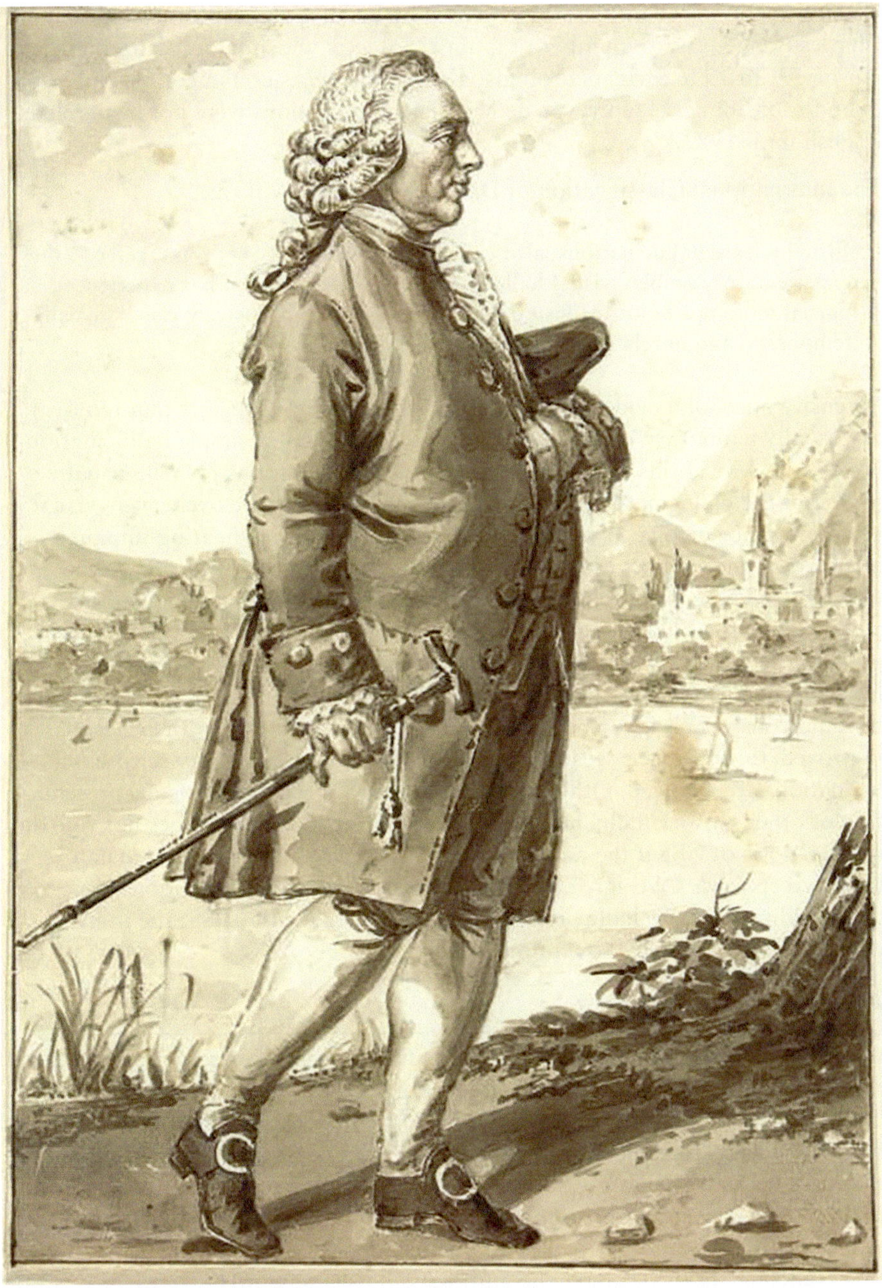

Figure 8.1 Watercolor painting of Charles Bonnet dressed in 17th-century attire. The Elisha Whittelsey Collection, The Elisha Whittelsey Fund, 1949.

his own vision loss. This was documented by his biographer who stated that Charles Bonnet saw "a number of fantastic objects which he recognized as illusory."[12] In 1936 Swiss neurologist Georges de Morsier named this condition in honor of Bonnet.[13] However, de Morsier's publications were not available in English until 1982.[14]

The International Classification of Diseases 11 defines CBS as:

> Visual release hallucinations, also called Charles Bonnet Syndrome, refer to the experience of complex visual hallucinations in a person who has experienced partial or complete loss of vision. Hallucinations are exclusively visual, usually temporary, and unrelated to mental and behavioral disorders.[15]

Extensive anecdotal evidence from CBS support groups suggests that removal of "usually temporary" is warranted. The contribution of simple hallucinations is also not clear in this definition.[16] The standard definitions for CBS usually state that the hallucinatory experiences of the condition are exclusively visual and should not involve any of the other senses.[5] Yet, some hearing-impaired members of the support groups have reported auditory input during a CBS experience. These patients are experiencing auditory release hallucinations secondary to their hearing loss, sometimes misnamed "auditory CBS".[17, 18] These particular individuals of the CBS support group have deficits in both vision and hearing; therefore, they are experiencing the release phenomena for both senses simultaneously. This is further confirmed by the fact that when their hearing is improved, through their wearing of the hearing aid, the auditory release hallucinations are resolved. Other authors believe that the simultaneous presentation of other sensory hallucinations with visual hallucinations does not rule out the diagnosis of CBS if the patient retains insight into the nongenuine nature of their perceptions.[19] We agree that other sensory release hallucinations, especially auditory release hallucinations, can be present with CBS if the individual comprehends that these perceptions are not real.

Anecdotal Evidence

One of the authors of this chapter (GMC) has convened a weekly support group for the past five years, bringing together individuals with CBS and their families. This has garnered information from over 150 contacts that is not detailed in formal studies. The referrals originated from patient internet research and contact with CBS information resources in the U.S.A., United Kingdom, Australia, and Canada. The support group prefers the word "images" to the more pejorative term "hallucinations." To be respectful to the actual individuals who have this syndrome, in this chapter the authors will use the word "images" instead of visual hallucinations.

Need for Differential Diagnosis

Suspicion that CBS has appeared in a person with a significant visual impairment should not prevent examination for an alternative diagnosis.[20] Briefly investigating for dementia, psychosis, and depression, by using tools such as the Montreal Cognitive Assessment-Blind, [21] the Brief Psychiatric Rating Scale, [22] and the Geriatric Depression Scale[23] respectively, could identify the need for further assessment. Conditions such as Parkinsons, Lewy Body Dementia, migraine aura, cortical insult and urinary tract infection may all cause visual images. The impact of prescribed medications and patient social milieu should also be considered.

One of the chapter authors (GMC) has worked with a few individuals with sight loss who adamantly insist that they are not visually impaired or blind. They may be mistaking CBS images for the return of real vision. People with Anton's Syndrome, which is usually the result of cortical insult, may give a rationale for sight-related difficulties that can sound like confabulation or delusion.[24] Determining if CBS is the cause of this belief or other causes will require careful discernment. [25]

Incidence, Prevalence, Age and Visual Acuity

Fear by patients of being diagnosed with dementia or psychosis makes it difficult to conduct CBS research. Research subject acquisition for CBS studies are hampered due to underreporting of the condition at every age. Research in the CBS population is typically a retrospective convenience sample formed by eye center records, or a survey given to a target group.[26]

Incidence is the risk of new occurrences in a specific population. The insidious nature of CBS development can make an accurate onset date after loss of vision difficult for patients to confirm. The incidence of CBS has been recorded in the literature to be as low as 0.5% and as high as 40%, depending on the patient population.[27, 28] An Australian study suggested that the average age at which people are diagnosed with CBS is 77.7 years old, with a range from 75 to 80.[29] Prevalence is the number of new and existing cases in a particular population at a specific time interval. A small prevalence study of younger ophthalmology patients aged 18 to 60 drawn from existing records found an average age of 39.4 in those with CBS.[30] Age is often mistaken as a risk factor for CBS, but children who had sight from birth to approximately age seven and then lost it, can develop CBS.[31]

As the population ages, CBS becomes more prevalent, more cases exist. This is due to the progression of chronic eye diseases such as macular degeneration, glaucoma, cataract, etc. (Table 8.1).[32] As a result, there may be an overrepresentation of older people with both macular and other ocular diseases in such studies.[5]

Vision loss is a necessary criterion for the diagnosis of CBS. Exactly how much vision loss does not appear to have been definitively determined, but both the loss of visual acuity and field of vision contribute.[33] In one large European study it was found that in their patient cohort the vision in the better-seeing eye was 20/40 or less.[34] This 20/40 threshold was confirmed in a different study.[35] It has

Table 8.1 Ophthalmic disease associated with visual hallucinations

• Age-Related Macular Degeneration
• Diabetic Retinopathy
• Glaucoma
• Cataracts
• Corneal Disease
• Enucleation
• Optic Neuritis/Optic Atrophy
• Central Retinal Artery Occlusion
• Retinitis Pigmentosa
• Macular Photocoagulation/Translocation
• Leber's Hereditary Optic Neuropathy
• Ocular Trauma
• AIDS and Cytomegalovirus Retinitis
• Choroideremia
• Cortex Pathology

With permission from Zerilli-Zavgorodni T, Bisighini S, Charles Bonnet Syndrome: comprehensive review providing an optometric approach to diagnosis and management. *Optom Vis Perf.* 2014;2(1):26–38.

also been proposed that CBS can occur with loss of vision in only one eye and normal vision remaining in the fellow eye.[36] One study found that reduced/low contrast sensitivity levels were strongly associated with CBS imagery.[37] Clearly, the final word on this matter has not yet been written. One factor that is constant is that the risk of developing CBS increases with worsening vision.[35] It also appears that the threshold of vision loss necessary to develop CBS is unique to every individual.

Perception

Perception refers to how the world around us is interpreted and understood, while reality is the actual state of things as they exist independent of our interpretations. Although our perceptions can shape our experiences, they do not always align with objective reality. Perception is not just seeing, however. Visual perception is moderated by past visual memories, current stimulation, and predictions of the future.[38] Our senses provide bottom-up information to our brains. Our brains moderate this in a top-down manner that creates its version of reality to our consciousness. Awareness of this edited reality arrives 50 to 100 milliseconds after the fact. During these milliseconds, multiple brain areas, forming a template or cognitive map from past experience and prior belief, generate predictions of reality from bottom-up visual stimulus.[39] This top-down prediction (brain influences the data being captured) forms a template of expected visual stimulus that is compared to bottom-up (gathering information from the periphery and funneling it to the brain) visual input.[40] In the absence of bottom-up visual input, the prediction becomes the perception of the CBS image.

Prior belief can override visual information in the process of object recognition.[16, 41] When there is a discrepancy between belief and visual input, the brain typically weighs belief as most accurate. This can result in images in which objective evidence is ignored. The influence of prior belief as a top-down trigger for CBS images is however being debated.[42, 43]

What is perceived in CBS patients bears no resemblance to reality in severe vision loss. Those with residual vision will blend prediction and prior beliefs with whatever they actually see. In some patients, CBS can block residual vision, allowing only the CBS image.

Image Content

Complex images caused by CBS are more likely to be reported since they may be more worrisome to an individual than simple or elementary images such as natural or intense colors, lights, shadows, and various shapes such as stars and patterns.[35] A single color filling the visual field has been reported.[5] People (complex imagery), followed by geometric patterns (simple imagery), are the most frequent images reported by CBS patients with end-stage age-related macular degeneration.[44] According to a study, 72% of patients with end-stage age-related macular degeneration see colored images.[44] Typically, images seen by most CBS patients may return and even be multiplied at varying time intervals; they are usually stereotyped.[5] If a different image is substituted, it is usually placed into a similar situation.[5] The imagery of CBS presents itself with endless variations.[9]

Details are vivid in complex images compared to simple images. Coming from the brain rather than the eye, these non-retinal images can appear in better focus and fill more of the visual field than is possible given the person's remaining vision. Images may be incomplete in that some of these images, for example of people, are missing body parts or have a distorted appearance. One of the hallmark features of some of the images in CBS is seeing people, objects and structures that appear reduced in size. This effect is termed Lilliputian, after the islanders of Lilliput in Jonathan Swift's *Gulliver's Travels*.[3] On the other hand, some CBS patients will see giants or significantly enlarged objects.[4] Charles Lullin experienced examples of both types of imagery. Faces and immersive images (whole environment) are usually not recognizable as these images come from semantic rather than autobiographical visual memory. The content is not recognized by the patient. These images have been occasionally labeled as proto-objects or proto-images.[2] The imagery and its surrounding scene are not personal, in contrast to those of the patient's imagination or recollection.[2] Another set of images, which occur in up to 25% of CBS patients, are text hallucinations.[2] These can include printed or handwritten words, words which appear to be in a foreign language, numbers, musical notes and symbols; they are all, however, uniformly incomprehensible no matter how closely the patient studies them.

CBS images vary for each person and throughout the day. One support group member calling this a "cast change" in the theater of the mind. Images may be static or moving and may appear to interact with the real environment. Images have been described as floating, moving collectively as one unit (without internal change) or dynamic (with internal movement).[9, 45, 46] Cartoon-like images, or even specific cartoon characters such as Bart Simpson or Minnie Mouse, can occur in either color or black and white.[3, 47] Animals may look like a typical specimen or may have fantastic combinations of highlights. Household pets may increase in number. Animals normally only seen in the wild and not typically thought of as pets will also appear. Images of insects are common.

In most instances, images of people are solid and present as being real; occasionally, however, they may appear two-dimensional.[2] The human images may be distorted with bizarre incongruities. Human images may wear either familiar uniforms or elaborate fanciful and fantastical costumes with a strong disposition to the exotic, often from an earlier time period.[2] They may be engaged in any type of human behavior. Images of people may appear to be moving their mouths and talking, but the image is always silent with no sound emanating. Occasionally, an image will appear to look at the patient; yet more often there is no attempt at the image to interact with the patient. The images remain silent and neutral, not having any personal connection with the patient.[34] Patients may perceive images of themselves (autoscopia), sometimes at earlier stages of their lives.[5] Threatening gestures and behavior by these images have also been reported by support group members. This is not the norm since, in most cases, the images are non-threatening and more often even quite pleasant; in some instances, however, patients may find them irritating and anxiety-inducing.[14, 34] Teunisse et al. found that, in their study of 60 patients with CBS, 28% experienced considerable distress from their images even though 77% felt the images lacked a personal meaning.[48] In his book, Leschziner introduces a person with CBS who has discovered that the images she sees correlate directly to her emotional state.[3] When she is sad, angry or anxious (her "down emotions"), she perceives "zombie faces, devils and dogs," but when she is happy and relaxed she perceives "floaty colors and bubbles and unicorns."[3] Her zombie faces are "cartoonish with blood dripping from their eyes and gnarly teeth."[3] Although she was frightened by them, she always retained insight and knew they were not real.[3]

People with CBS have reported seeing an immersive or 360° environment. They may perceive that they are in a different house, building, or landscape. Some support group members report this occurs upon waking. This has been documented by other researchers as the state of drowsy wakefulness.[49] These images have also been reported to appear at dusk in familiar surroundings of the patients' homes; most patients cannot identify any specific activity in which they were involved that brought forth the images.[34]

Episodes

Episodes are involuntary and can be startling, beginning without warning or aura as seen in migraines. Perception of images with eyes open or closed varies among patients. CBS images may last for seconds, hours, or a full day and can be described as vivid, detailed, and organized.[50, 51] Episodes can be chronic, persisting weeks or months with varying intensity, or sporadic, often ceasing for days or weeks.

Onset and Duration

The onset and progression of CBS varies from individual to individual. Support group members have reported CBS onset immediately occurring upon significant sight loss, or beginning a number of weeks after their vision loss; in one instance a member's CBS appeared after six years of total blindness. The most common progression is the initial appearance of simple images, accompanied somewhat later by complex images. Both simple and complex images may occur during a single day, either separately or concurrently.

Questionnaires completed by United Kingdom Macular Society members identified 492 people with CBS, 75% of which had experienced the condition for five or more years.[51] This calls into question the early research, which had given 18 months as the typical duration of CBS.[52, 53] Some support group members have experienced CBS for decades, indicating that not all these visual hallucinations dissipate over time as has been frequently assumed.

Insight

The patient has at least partial insight that the images are not real. This conviction may waver during the course of a single potential episode. Insight into the unreality of CBS images improves over time. With information and support, nearly all people with CBS will see the images more as an inconvenience than an invasion. This assertion also helps to decrease the frequency of CBS as well as the level of disturbance.

A few people with CBS, however, will insist on the reality of the images. These patients in particular may flee, fight, or fawn because of increasing anxiety.[54] Injuries have occurred due to attempts to attack or escape the images. Caregivers have reported that individuals with CBS in their care will try to feed or otherwise make the images comfortable.

Even though the image is silent, the patient with CBS may just "know" or intuit what the image wants them to know. Acting on image-directed instructions has been reported. This includes modifying the patient's living situation or following the image through doors. In the case of these individuals, safety should always be the first consideration. Following the experience of an image that is frightening, the CBS patient may begin to experience anticipatory anxiety. Symptoms of a panic attack may be present during episodes and should be assessed.[55] Some patients may need referral to formal behavioral therapy such as cognitive behavior therapy for this anxiety caused by their medical condition.[56]

Triggers

Some situations are more likely to give rise to images. Riding in a car and grocery shopping are frequently mentioned. Dr. Oliver Sacks has labeled this visual movement as "optic flow" and felt that it was especially provocative in producing images in CBS patients.[2] The induced images may be plausible and in context; more often, however, they involve rather elaborate scenes which are not necessarily even remotely related to what is actually physically present. The patient can "see" these elaborate scenes, whether they keep their eyes open or closed.[2] According to Gilmour, et al., the most common triggering factors were: level of illumination (dim/bright) (20%); fatigue (8%); physical and mental stressors (4%) and social or physical isolation and loneliness (2%).[35] The loneliness and isolation experienced during the recent COVID-19 pandemic quarantine seemed to increase hallucinations in some people with CBS.[57] Fully sighted people who are isolated in solitary confinement are known to experience hallucinations even without a visual loss.[58] From a theoretical point of view, it seems possible that reduced sensory stimulation, as in the case of living in isolation or having a lack of social contact, would trigger CBS images.[59]

Patients who are exhausted from CBS images which are disturbing their sleep are more likely to see an exacerbation of images. It is also shown that drowsiness increases the likelihood of hallucination, suggesting that the reticular activating system plays a role in visual hallucinations. All hallucinations are more likely in low light situations such as dusk. Physicians may mistakenly interpret this as the "sundowning" seen in dementia patients, but this is only a coincidence.

Inhibitors

Optimizing visual function as well as clinician awareness, compassion and reassurance for the patient that their mental health is intact are the primary prevention modalities for CBS.[20, 60] Rapid blinking of the eyes, saccadic eye movements, and briefly closing one's eyes have long been recommended as a coping mechanism for CBS.[34, 61]

Websites offer many suggestions regarding coping with CBS images.[62]

- Change or begin an activity
- Change lighting (usually increase illumination)
- Attempt to touch image
- Engagement with others
- Support groups
- Seek counseling to deal with emotions regarding CBS

The website CharlesBonnet.com suggests not taking a victim role, trying to regain one's quality of life that they had before CBS onset, and seeking out family, friends, and support groups who take an interest in your experiences.[63] Challenge the images and yourself by attempting to touch them. Gain blindness skills and confidence through involvement with private and state blind organizations.

Treatment

Optimizing visual function through the use of refraction to attain best-corrected spectacle visual acuity, visual aids or other low-vision devices and referral to a low-vision specialist to help evaluate and prescribe these aids and devices is recommended. Pursuing promising surgical procedures such as cataract extraction with intraocular lens implantation, laser photocoagulation for proliferative diabetic retinopathy, or intravitreal anti-vascular endothelial growth factor injections for patients with macular degeneration may improve visual function and halt symptom progression.[60] One of the authors of this chapter (LS) has "cured" CBS in select patients with appropriate and needed ophthalmic surgical/procedural intervention which improved their vision. In analogous sensory deprivation research, sighted subjects stopped experiencing hallucinations when the blindfold was removed.[64]

A review of potential hallucination-inducing medications that the patient may unknowingly be taking and blood lab testing for underlying vitamin deficiencies or concurrent infections should be performed by a primary care physician.[65] There is currently no definitive medical treatment for CBS. A person with CBS has a medical problem due to their sight impairment. This medical problem can secondarily engender a problem with their mental health. Management primarily involves educating patients and providing reassurance about the benign nature of the condition. Medications like anticonvulsants or anti-psychotics have been used in severe cases, though with limited success.[66] Cognitive behavioral therapy and metacognitive therapy has shown promise with some support group members.

First contact is almost always a call to a help line or support group provider regarding CBS. That contact will be with a paraprofessional who is knowledgeable regarding CBS but not trained in mental health. Research on cognitive behavior therapy suggests that paraprofessionals may be trained to deliver a preliminary intervention by telephone.[67] This should be augmented by referral to a local therapist who can assess for any panic symptoms. The only contraindication is that in general, some behavior therapists may be unfamiliar with CBS.

As stated in Chapter 1, the Foundation for Fighting Blindness has developed therapist training in working with a person who is visually impaired and has partnered with a nationwide telehealth service.[68] This is a promising strategy to deal with patients who cannot drive to therapy meetings.

Charles Bonnet Syndrome Theories

1. Most common: ocular pathology

   Subject acquisition in CBS studies is difficult due to underreporting of the condition. As a result, there may be an overrepresentation of individuals with retinal and macular diseases, especially in the more recent studies.[29] Any injury to the visual tract that causes significant vision loss such as disease sequalae, stroke, or trauma may cause CBS.

2. Deafferentation

   Deafferentation theory suggests that compensation for decreased sensory input, due to loss of vision, lowers the activation threshold of visual pathways in individuals with CBS. This can result in cortical hyperexcitability or reduction of sensory inhibitory networks that are ordinarily in force.[69] Functional neuroimaging studies have found areas corresponding to normal vision hyperexcited producing a CBS image.[70, 71]

3. Release Theory

   Sensory deprivation and bereavement studies have shown that individuals without visual impairment may experience visual images.[72, 73] This suggests that loss of visual input can reduce possible hallucinatory perception to a type of baseline memory. The generic visual memory releases to one's perception visual memories unrelated to experience, which ordinarily serve to speed recognition in normal vision. This generic visual memory is known as semantic visual memory. This may mean that the loss of input, rather than any physical damage in vision loss, is the actual cause of the image.

4. Irritative Theory

   Irritative theory states that visual hallucinations may be caused by spontaneous epileptiform discharge from vascular dysfunction, cranial arteritis or other lesions. The variety of visual images argue against this theory as visual pathways without injury or insult are active. This is also not supported by neuroimaging.[60]

REFERENCES

1. Rosenbaum R, Why Oliver Sacks is one of the great modern adventurers: The neurologist's latest investigations of the mind explore the mystery of hallucinations – including his own. *Smithsonian Mag.* 2012 December. [cited 2025 September 8] https://www.smithsonianmag.com/science-nature/why-oliver-sacks-is-one-of-the-great-modern-adventurers-134428056/.
2. Sacks O, *Hallucinations*. New York: Alfred A Knopf; 2012: 3–33.
3. Leschziner G, *The Man Who Tasted Words*. New York: St Martin's Press; 2022: 49–85.
4. De Morsier G, Le syndrome de Charles Bonnet: Hallucinations visuelles des vieillards sans déficience mentale. *Ann Méd Psychol.* 1967;125:677–702.
5. Menon GJ et al., Complex visual hallucinations in the visually impaired. *Surv Ophthalmol.* 2003;48(1):58–72.
6. Chisholm H, ed., Bonnet, Charles. *Encycl Brit.* Vol. 4 (11th ed.). Cambridge: Cambridge Univ Press; 1911:211.
7. Rigato E et al., *Evo Edu Outreach.* 2013. https://doi.org/10.1186/1936-6434-6-18
8. Bonnet C, *Essai Analytique sur les Facultés de L'âme*, 2nd edn. Copenhagen and Geneva: Philibert; 1769:176–7.
9. Draaisma D, *Disturbances of the Mind*. Cambridge: Cambridge Univ Press; 2009:11–39.
10. Berrios GE, *The History of Mental Symptoms: Descriptive Psychopathology Since the Nineteenth Century*. Cambridge: Cambridge Univ Press; 1996:42.

11. Bonnet C, *Analytical Essay on the Faculties of the Soul*, Gaukroger S (trans.). Oxford: Oxford Univ Press; 2022:234.
12. Levêque de Pouilly JS, *Éloge de Charles Bonnet*. Lausanne: Henbach; 1794:120–1.
13. De Morsier G, Les automatismes visuels. Hallucinations retrochiasmatiques. *Schweiz Med Wochenschr.* 1936;66:700–8.
14. Damas-Mora J et al., The Charles Bonnet syndrome in perspective. *Psychol Med.* 1982;12(2):251–61.
15. World Health Organization, *International Statistical Classification of Diseases and Related Health Problems* (11th ed.) [Internet]. *Int Classif Dis 11th Rev*. 2019. Available from: https://icd.who.int/
16. Jones L et al., From research to action: Recommendations for Charles Bonnet syndrome care and policy. *BMJ Open Ophthalmol* [Internet]. 2025 May 1 [cited 2025 May 13];10(1):e002009–9. Available from: https://bmjophth.bmj.com/content/10/1/e002009
17. Restrepo-Carvajal LC et al., *Acta Neurol Belg*. 2025. https://doi.org/10.1007/s13760-025-02824-w
18. Sacks O, *Musicophilia*. New York: Vintage Books; 2008:57,195–6.
19. Hori H et al., Charles Bonnet syndrome with auditory hallucinations: A diagnostic dilemma. *Psychopathology.* 2001;34:164–6.
20. Kelson T et al., Out of sight, am I losing my mind? A case report on visual release hallucinations – Charles Bonnet syndrome. *Psychiatry Res Case Rep*. 2022;1(2):1–3.
21. Nasreddine ZS et al., The Montreal Cognitive Assessment, MoCA: A brief screening tool for mild cognitive impairment. *J Am Geriatr Soc.* 2005;53(4):695–9.
22. Stojan B et al., Factor structure of the brief psychiatric rating scale-expanded among outpatients with psychotic disorders in five Southeast European countries: Evidence for five factors. *Front Psychiatry.* 2023;14(14):1–9.
23. Devita M et al., Recognizing depression in the elderly: Practical guidance and challenges for clinical management. *Neuropsychiatr Dis Treat.* 2022;18(1):2867–80.
24. Atallah O et al., *J Clin Neurosci*. 2024. https://doi.org/10.1016/j.jocn.2024.01.014
25. Kisling L et al., Prevention strategies [Internet]. *Natl Libr Med*. StatPearls Publishing; 2023. Available from: https://www.ncbi.nlm.nih.gov/books/NBK537222/
26. Baffour-Awuah KA et al., The missing pieces: An investigation into the parallels between Charles Bonnet, phantom limb, and tinnitus syndromes. *Ther Adv Ophthalmol*. 2024;16:1–21.
27. Shiraishi Y et al., The rarity of Charles Bonnet syndrome. *J Psychiatr Res.* 2004;38:207–13.
28. Abbott EJ et al., Visual loss and visual hallucinations in patients with age-related macular degeneration (Charles Bonnet syndrome). *Invest Ophthalmol Vis Sci.* 2007;48:1416–23.

29. Vukicevic M et al., *Clin Exp Ophthalmol.* 2008. https://doi.org/10.1111/j.1442-9071.2008.01814.x. PMID: 18983551
30. Karagöl A, *Psychiatr Danub.* 2021. PMID: 34718287
31. Elflein HM et al., Charles Bonnet's syndrome: Not only a condition of the elderly. *Graefes Arch Clin Exp Ophthalmol.* 2016;254(8):1637–42.
32. Rojas LC et al., *Charles Bonnet syndrome* [Internet]. StatPearls Publishing; 2023 [cited 2025 Jul 28]. Available from: https://www.ncbi.nlm.nih.gov/books/NBK585133
33. Jan T et al., *West J Emerg Med.* 2012. https://doi.org/10.5811/westjem.2012.7.12891. PMID: 23357937; PMCID: PMC3555593
34. Teunisse RJ et al., The Charles Bonnet syndrome: A large prospective study in The Netherlands. A study of the prevalence of the Charles Bonnet syndrome and associated factors in 500 patients attending the University Department of Ophthalmology at Nijmegen. *Br J Psychiatry.* 1995;166(2):254–7.
35. Gilmour G et al., An examination of the relationship between low vision and Charles Bonnet syndrome. *Can J Ophthalmol.* 2009;44:49–52.
36. Forte G et al., *Ophthalmic Physiol Opt.* 2025. https://doi.org/10.1111/opo.13481
37. Jackson ML et al., Contrast sensitivity and visual hallucinations in patients referred to a low vision rehabilitation clinic. *Br J Ophthalmol.* 2007;91:296–8.
38. Pearson J et al., Phantom perception: Voluntary and involuntary nonretinal vision. *Trends Cogn Sci.* 2015;19(5):278–84.
39. Franconeri SL et al., *Trends Cogn Sci.* 2013. https://doi.org/10.1016/j.tics.2013.01.010
40. Kok P et al., *J Cogn Neurosci.* 2014. https://doi.org/10.1162/jocn_a_00562. PMID: 24392894
41. Del Rio M et al., The mechanisms underlying conditioning of phantom percepts differ between those with hallucinations and synesthesia. *Sci Rep.* 2024;14:5607:1–10.
42. Powers AR et al., Hallucinations as top-down effects on perception. *Biol Psychiatry Cogn Neurosci Neuroimaging.* 2016;1(5):393–400.
43. Schmid FR et al., Explanatory power by vagueness: Challenges to the strong prior hypothesis on hallucinations exemplified by the Charles-Bonnet syndrome. *Conscious Cogn* [Internet]. 2024 January 1 [cited 2024 Jan 23];117:103620. Available from: https://www.sciencedirect.com/science/article/pii/S1053810023001575
44. Khan JC et al., Charles Bonnet syndrome in age-related macular degeneration: The nature and frequency of images in subjects with end-stage disease. *Ophthalmic Epidemiol.* 2008;15:202–8.
45. Fernandez A et al., The Charles Bonnet syndrome: A review. *J Nerv Ment Dis.* 1997;185:195–200.
46. Schultz G et al., The Charles Bonnet syndrome: Phantom visual images. *Perception.* 1991;20:809–25.

47. Francis G et al., Simulations of induced visual scene fading with boundary offset and filling-in. *Vis Res.* 2012;62:181–91.
48. Teunisse RJ et al., Visual hallucinations in psychologically normal people: Charles Bonnet's syndrome. *Lancet.* 1996;347:794–7.
49. Ffytche DH, Visual hallucinations and the Charles Bonnet syndrome. *Curr Psychiatry Rep.* 2005;7:168–79.
50. Teeple RC et al., Visual hallucinations. *Prim Care Companion J Clin Psychiatry* [Internet]. 2009;11(1):26–32. Available from: https://pmc.ncbi.nlm.nih.gov/articles/PMC2660156/
51. Cox TM et al., Negative outcome Charles Bonnet syndrome. *Br J Ophthalmol* [Internet]. 2014;98(9):1236–9. Available from: https://bjo.bmj.com/content/98/9/1236
52. Cumming AL et al., Charles Bonnet syndrome: A literature review. *Br J Ophthalmol.* 2011;95(8):1106–11.
53. Jackson ML et al., The natural history of the Charles Bonnet syndrome: Do the hallucinations go away? *Eye.* 2010;24:1303–4.
54. Holroyd S et al., Visual hallucinations in patients from an ophthalmology clinic and medical clinic population. *J Nerv Ment Dis.* 1994;182:273–6.
55. Raju NN et al., Clinical practice guidelines for assessment and management of anxiety and panic disorders in emergency setting. *Indian J Psychiatry.* 2023 Feb;65(2):181–5.
56. American Psychiatric Association, *Diagnostic and Statistical Manual of Mental Disorders*, 5th edn. Arlington, VA: American Psychiatric Publishing; 2013:210.
57. Jones L et al., Exacerbation of visual hallucinations in Charles Bonnet syndrome due to the social implications of COVID-19. *BMJ Open Ophthalmol.* 2021;6(1):e000670.
58. Reiter K et al., Psychological distress in solitary confinement: Symptoms, severity, and prevalence in the United States, 2017–2018. *Am J Public Health* [Internet]. 2020;110(S1):S56–62. Available from: https://ajph.aphapublications.org/doi/full/10.2105/AJPH.2019.305375
59. Zerilli-Zavgorodni T et al., Charles Bonnet syndrome: Comprehensive review providing an optometric approach to diagnosis and management. *Optom Vis Perf.* 2014;2:26–38.
60. Zaman M, Skorin L, The ophthalmologist's map to Charles Bonnet syndrome. *Eyes On Eyecare.* 2023. https://eyesoneyecare.com/resources/ophthalmologists-map-to-charles-bonnet-syndrome/
61. Issa BA et al., Charles Bonnet syndrome, management with simple behavioral technique. *J Neurosci Rural Pract.* 2013;4(1):63–5.
62. Charles Bonnet syndrome: Visual hallucinations caused by sight loss. Understanding [Internet]. [cited 2025 Jul 28]. Available from: https://hadleyhelps.org/sites/default/files/2024-03/Understanding_Charles_Bonnet_Syndrome.pdf
63. Bonnet C, Charles Bonnet syndrome information [Internet]. 2022 [cited 2025 Jul 28]. Available from: https://charlesbonnet.com/

64. Merabet LB et al., Visual hallucinations during prolonged blindfolding in sighted subjects. *J Neuro-Ophthalmol.* 2004;24(2):109–13.
65. Ffytche DH, Visual hallucination and illusion disorders: A clinical guide. *Adv Clin Neurosci Rehabil.* 2004;4:16–8.
66. Alamri SH, A low dose of risperidone resolved Charles Bonnet syndrome after an unsuccessful trial of quetiapine: A case report. *Neuropsychiatr Dis Treat.* 2018;14:809–11.
67. Somer E et al., Brief cognitive-behavioral phone-based intervention targeting anxiety about the threat of attack: A pilot study. *Behav Res Ther.* 2005;43:669–79.
68. Personal communication Peter Ginsberg, Foundation Fighting Blindness 6/11/25.
69. Ffytche DH, Visual hallucinations in eye disease. *Curr Opin Neurol.* 2009;22:28–35.
70. Ffytche DH et al., The anatomy of conscious vision: An fMRI study of visual hallucinations. *Nat Neurosci* [Internet]. 1998 Dec 1 [cited 2020 Jun 21];1(8):738–42. Available from: https://pubmed.ncbi.nlm.nih.gov/10196592/
71. Hahamy A et al., How do the blind 'see'? The role of spontaneous brain activity in self-generated perception. *Brain.* 2021;144:340–53.
72. Eperjesi F, Visual hallucinations in Charles Bonnet syndrome. In: Larøi F, Aleman A, eds. *Hallucinations: A Guide to Treatment and Management.* Oxford: Oxford Univ Press; 2010:303–22.
73. Castelnovo A et al., Post-bereavement hallucinatory experiences: A critical overview of population and clinical studies. *J Affect Disord.* 2015;186:266–74.

Chapter 9

LOW VISION

Karen Squier, Charlie Saccarelli, Denise Goodwin and Meagan Chapman

Low Vision Examination

Introduction

Patients with visual impairment are referred for a low vision examination to assist with improving function, safety and independence via an evaluation by a practitioner who performs an assessment of one's impairment related to ocular disease. The low vision practitioner can recommend assistive devices, compensatory strategies and community resources aimed at improving quality of life. Through these examinations, hallucinations, such as those seen in Charles Bonnet Syndrome (CBS), may be mentioned and thus it's important to understand their impact and how to counsel patients on their presence and meaning.[1] Vision loss is disruptive to daily living, as is CBS, and attempts to rehabilitate these difficulties should be attempted.[2]

Case History

The case history of a low vision examination is the first opportunity for the eye care clinician (ECC) to uncover visual challenges the patient is experiencing, probe emotional difficulties and assess the prognosis for rehabilitation. The low vision case history is an extension of the traditional medical history and allows the ECC to delve further regarding the impact an ocular or systemic disease has had on the patient's quality of life and daily activities.

Knowing a patient's hobbies and which ones they have had to stop, employment status and daily scheduled activities are valuable. The ECC can then focus on opportunities for visual enhancement and the patient's motivation for functional improvement beyond visual acuity. Patients with visual impairment may share socio-economic challenges or personal goals of seeking employment. Early vision loss may contribute to unemployment, and identifying ways to enhance vision can allow someone to maintain or return to employment.[3]

It is imperative for the ECC to ask this line of questioning, even though it deviates from the traditional medical history questions.

Activities of Daily Living (ADLs) and Instrumental Activities for Independent Living (IADLs) are each important considerations of patients who have experienced vision loss.[4] ADLs include activities of self-care, grooming or hygiene such as bathing, dressing and eating. IADLs are more complex activities that one needs to accomplish when living in a community, such as financial management,

DOI: 10.1201/9781003633365-9

driving and meal preparation. With worsening vision, both ADLs and IADLs become more difficult to perform and thus need modifications for independent management or assistance from another person. Safety and health concerns grow as vision loss worsens. While there has been no identified correlation of CBS impacting ADLs, worsening vision loss may correlate to an increase in hallucinations as well as an increased difficulties in performing independent tasks.

Previous low vision device history as well as services should be assessed to help with streamlining the examination. Patients who have used low vision devices in the past, but have abandoned them, should be queried as to their reasons for acting in this way. Device abandonment has been found to be correlated with devices that fail to improve quality of life or in patients with peripheral vision loss.[5, 6] This speaks to the importance of a thorough history, careful device selection and training along with collaborating with appropriate rehabilitation professionals to ensure a positive impact.

Another consideration is the patient's use of consumer technology. Use of smart technology amongst visually impaired patients has increased. Smart technology, such as accessibility options and apps, can transform a smartphone or tablet into a functional device that can help with communication, navigation, ADLs and IADLs. One growing area of development is the use of artificial intelligence in the low vision community. Apps that offer artificial intelligence for identifying objects or provide guidance with micronavigation challenges are an emerging area of development in the low vision world.[7]

Changes in visual function can impact driving performance. Patients with vision loss may no longer meet their local government's requirements for independent driving. This may result in individuals having difficulty with getting to appointments or limited social activity and interaction. In some individuals, driving cessation can lead to depression as loss of independence can be difficult to accept. This may result in denial, and a person with vision loss may continue to drive despite counseling by their ECC. Patients are often hesitant to bring up driving for fear of loss of licensure. Ask direct and non-judgmental questions about their driving status and access to reliable transportation. For patients who are visually impaired, but are still legal to drive, discussion on how their vision loss impacts driving safety is important. Performance in inclement weather, preferred routes, and response to sunlight should be part of the questions asked during the case history. It is important for the ECC to know their local driving laws so they can counsel their patients in terms of how their vision aligns with driving standards and possible challenges in driving due to loss of contrast or visual blur.

Conditions that cause peripheral field loss are known instigators of mobility issues. Conditions that create asymmetric vision loss may also create difficulties with judging depth or ambulating on uneven surfaces. Patients with poor contrast sensitivity should also be queried as to difficulties with mobility.

Some patients have difficulties with daily tasks like reading mail or nutrition labels. Questions about adaptations given their current vision can help glean their level of functional vision. For instance, if a person needed to see a nutrition label, do they use a magnifier or ask someone to do that task for them? Another area would be staying on top of current events. Does one read a newspaper on paper or reads while using an app on their tablet? Do they read articles or skim the headlines? Or, instead, do they listen to the evening news? Questions about current function should be detailed enough for the ECC to visualize how a patient is functioning in their home, and what challenges the patient has in their everyday life. This can help guide referrals and device selection. It is also helpful to review whether CBS symptoms increase or decrease in frequency with different tasks.

The case history for most medical examinations is problem-specific, while low vision case histories focus on functional challenges that the patient experiences and helps with creation of goals. Visual goals help drive the assistive device assessment for a patient. Uncovering the patient's goals is an opportunity to determine the patient's motivation and whether the patient has a realistic expectation for their visual rehabilitation.

During the case history, it is helpful to provide an opportunity to discuss whether a patient is experiencing CBS. As the clinician develops a rapport with the patient, the patient's comfort level with answering questions often increases. In order to reduce patient anxiety and defensiveness, it is helpful to frame questions about CBS in a manner that does not single out their experience, but rather demonstrates that it is a common situation amongst people with similar vision deficits. A questionnaire has been developed for gathering information about the type, frequency and associated challenges (Table 9.1).[8]

Emotional Status

Patients with visual impairment have a higher prevalence of emotional issues. For instance, patients with glaucoma have a higher prevalence of depression and anxiety, and additional comorbidities may also worsen mental health status.[9, 10] Changes in emotional status have been found to change the quality of hallucinations in patients with CBS.[8, 9]

Table 9.1 Clinical questionnaire for describing Charles Bonnet Hallucinations

What images are you seeing?
What is the frequency of the hallucinations?
How long does each episode last? Describe the onset of the hallucinations.
What are the lighting conditions at the time of a hallucinatory episode?
What are the conditions at the time of the hallucination?
Is there anything that you do that could make the hallucination stop?
How stressful are the hallucinations to you? Have you told anyone about the hallucinations?

Adapted With Permission from Vukicevic M, et al., *Clin Exp Ophthalmol.* 2008. doi:10.1111/j.1442-9071.2008.01814.x.

While emotional counseling is not part of the scope of practice for the ECC, it is important to address a visually impaired or blind individual's emotional status to ensure patients have appropriate psychological support and are referred for resources to improve their ability to adapt to their vision loss.[11, 12] Emotional status should be considered in discussions regarding outcomes as well as prognosis for rehabilitation success.

Visual Acuity Assessment

Proper selection of distance and near charts is crucial to assessing a patient's visual thresholds. Traditional projection and digital charts may not have the range of optotypes or presentation of standardized sizes to best assess patient's visual discrimination or functional vision, nor can they be moved closer to the visually impaired patient. Traditional distance charts that are commonly used in low vision examinations are the Early Treatment Diabetic Retinopathy Study Chart (ETDRS Chart), the Bailey-Lovie Chart, and the Feinbloom chart. The ETDRS Chart and Bailey-Lovie Charts each have a standardized presentation of optotypes that allows for a more accurate and repeatable assessment. Feinbloom low vision charts are handheld charts that offer a wide range of optotypes and can be moved closer to the patient but also easily moved into different fields of gaze to pick up peripheral vision for patients who are unable to efficiently use their eccentric viewing position. It is important during testing to keep the patient engaged to ensure symptomatic patients do not experience hallucinations during testing.

For near testing, many charts are available to assess a patient's near acuity and threshold. Most clinicians present charts that equate to the patient's goal; for instance, if a patient has a goal of reading a newspaper article, a continuous text chart should be used, while a single letter or single word might be more appropriate for spot reading. Coordination of eye movements may impact acuity thresholds and may show that patients have "worse" acuity on continuous text cards rather than single letter, so it's best to assess both before finalizing a device.

Entrance testing helps uncover additional features of a patient's functional vision. It is important to modify testing procedures to best capture a patient's visual abilities. Using larger targets for fixation and adjusting testing speed allows patients to participate more fully in testing. For patients who do not have functional levels of vision, testing is still important to rule out a neurologic defect. Giving verbal directions during pursuits or using doll's head movements can still allow the clinician the opportunity to determine if misalignment exists to rule out palsy or paresis.

Contrast Sensitivity

Contrast sensitivity loss is a measurement of the quality of vision, rather than visual discrimination, and is a standard test in a low vision examination. Contrast sensitivity can be impaired in different types of ocular disease such as glaucoma and macular degeneration, but can also be implicated in treatable anterior segment diseases such as dry eye and cataracts.[13, 14] Contrast sensitivity loss may be the cause of facial recognition difficulties, motion detection, and driving when high-contrast acuity charts do not reveal levels of functional loss despite patient complaints.[15]

Measuring contrast sensitivity loss clinically is often performed using standardized tests, such as Pelli-Robson or MARS contrast charts. Both charts have been shown to be reliable and repeatable. The Pelli-Robson chart is mounted on a wall at 1 meter and has 10 repeating letters in Sloan optotypes presented in triplets of descending contrast on 8 lines. The MARS card is a hand-held chart that is tested at a closer distance, between 40 and 60 centimeters. One primary difference from Pelli-Robson is that each letter on the MARS card has a decreasing contrast rather than triplets of letters. Both charts are reliable and repeatable tests that can be used clinically.[15] The information gleaned can provide guidance for referrals for in-home rehabilitation, device selection and orientation and mobility.

Refraction

Refraction of patients with visual impairments can be challenging, but it may provide a wealth of knowledge on the patient's true visual potential as well as qualify one for disability or community services. By understanding the potential impact of ocular and systemic pathology on the refractive error, the ECC has a starting point for correcting the refractive error.

Trial frame refraction is preferred as it allows patients to wear their initial refractive correction and to be able to adopt their natural viewing position. For patients with central scotomas from macular pathology or those that use a null point to dampen a nystagmus, trial frames allow for the patient to find their best viewing point during subjective testing. Traditional subjective testing also needs to be modified for patients with poor vision; a patient with best-corrected acuity of 20/200 would not be sensitive to the 0.25 diopter differences a phoropter offers. Adjusting lens choices to accommodate poor visual acuity is also key and allowing for best head posture is why trial frame is preferred.

Upon completion of refraction, the ECC has a best-corrected visual acuity. This is important in terms of determining the power of a device the patient needs for meeting their visual goals. It also assists the clinician in determining whether the patient qualifies for legal blindness or services based on their level of vision. Improving visual acuity has been demonstrated to reduce the frequency of CBS and thus refraction should also be assessed in these patients.[16]

Assistive Devices

Improvement in visual function has been shown to reduce the frequency and duration of hallucinations in patients experiencing CBS.[17, 18] Lighting and environment also needs to be considered.

For near viewing, several devices are available to achieve visual goals. Patients may have a goal that requires hands-free magnification, such as holding a textbook, compared to someone who needs to use a hand-held device for seeing a thermostat. Assistive devices continue to improve with changes in technology and the evolution of smart devices. Traditional low vision devices have optical design and may have built-in illumination. Newer assistive devices use touch screens, optical character recognition, and contrast-enhancing techniques.

Optical Devices

Microscopes

Microscopes are spectacle-mounted lenses that act as a converging system and allow the patient to hold print closer, thus creating a magnified retinal image. Microscopes can be single vision lenses, providing an improved field of view, or can take the form of a bifocal which only utilizes a segmented portion near the bottom of the lens.

Some of the difficulties using microscopes center on aberrations that are inherent to higher prescriptions. Lens treatments and coatings can help reduce the impact of these aberrations. Patients often have a difficult time with physically changing and maintaining their working distance from their habitual working distance.

Hand-held Magnifiers

Hand-held magnifiers are convex lenses that are held away from the spectacle plane, and when held near their focal point, create a magnified image. These devices are often used for spot reading, rather than prolonged reading. These magnifiers often have a built-in light source for illumination of their target print (Figure 9.1).

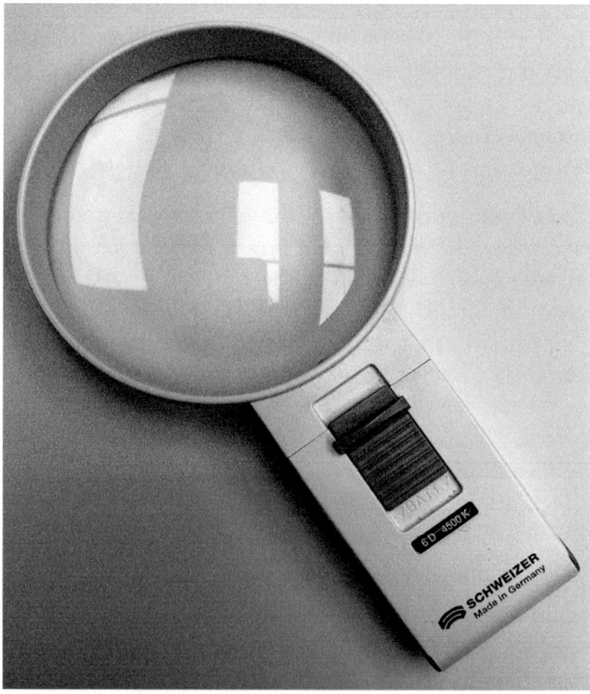

Figure 9.1 Hand-held magnifier.

Stand Magnifiers

Stand magnifiers are convex lenses that are mounted into a stand that allows for the lens to be supported without the patient needing to hold the device in free space. Many stand magnifiers have built-in lights to illuminate their object of interest. Reading stands and glare management help improve visual success with these devices.

Telescopes

Telescopes are optical devices that magnify objects at a distance. These devices are available in a wide range of powers and can be hand-held or spectacle-mounted. Spectacle-mounted telescopes can be used for driving depending on regional legislation. Telescopes can be difficult to use. Due to the reduced field of view, some individuals require significant training to use the device effectively. Additionally, hand-held telescopes can be difficult to use with patients who have tremors or weakness. Telescopes can be adapted for near use in the form of a telemicroscope to allow a longer working distance, while maintaining the same level of retinal magnification.

Electronic Devices

A large area of growth in low vision technology is the use of video magnifiers and closed circuit television to not only enlarge text but also change color settings to enhance contrast (Figure 9.2). Video magnifiers can be either portable or desktop versions which may suit a range of vocations and avocations. Given the larger screen size, patients can experience the level of magnification with a larger field of view. Additionally, the ability to alter contrast settings allows patients with moderate to severe levels of contrast loss to enhance their goal text to more functional levels of vision.

Additional low vision devices Figures 9.3a–e are available as an online resource in the Ancillary material section of Chapter 9.

Management of Field Loss

Hemianopia and Quadrantanopia Field Loss

Neurologic events, such as cerebral vascular accidents, neoplasm, aneurysms and brain trauma, create their own individual challenges with a patient's visual function.[19] Visual acuity, visual field or contrast sensitivity loss may occur if the visual pathways are involved. For patients with chiasmal or post-chiasmal lesions, visual field loss will be bilateral, and attention needs to be paid to the functional challenges field loss causes.[19, 20]

Most patients with solely post-chiasmal lesions will retain good visual acuity and normal contrast; when field loss is present, however, it can be debilitating.[21] Distance activities that require good mobility and spatial awareness are often significantly affected.[21] Driving and independent ambulation are both impacted, and the degree of impact may change depending on the environment one is in.[20] For instance, walking in a known area with little visual clutter, such as a neighborhood in a rural town, would likely be less difficult to manage compared

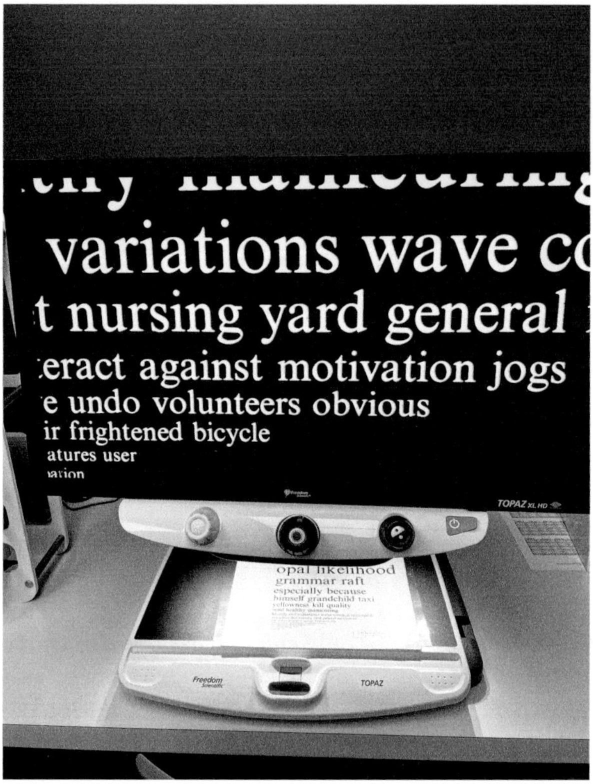

Figure 9.2 Closed circuit television.

to walking in a crowded aisle in a grocery store with a lot of visual stimulation. Reading can also be impacted by visual field loss; patients with left field loss may have difficulties finding the beginning of a line in an article of a newspaper. In patients with right field loss, difficulty knowing where the line ends can be a challenge. In addition to taking a good functional history of these patients, neurocognitive tests addressing spatial awareness and neglect help determine rehabilitation prognosis.

Rehabilitation of visual field loss first begins with identifying the type of visual field loss the patient has.[20] Kinetic visual fields, such as Goldmann visual fields, can provide an assessment of the visual field beyond the central 60 degrees. Automated visual fields can also provide critical information; however, they may be impacted if reaction time or executive function has been impacted by the neurologic event.[20]

Visual field rehabilitation for patients with hemianopia field loss typically is aimed at improving the patient's adaptation to the missing field by either optically expanding the visual field with prism or improving visual scanning to compensate for the missing field.[19] The success of either strategy will be impacted by cognition, motivation and status of the disease so it is important to provide realistic expectations to patients before rehabilitation begins.[20]

Prism placement provides an optical expansion of the patient's visual field with the goal of improving awareness in the missing field. The most common fitting strategy in recent years has been the use of Peli Prism Placement.[22] In this fitting scenario, base-out prism is placed above and below patient fixation allowing for good central visual acuity and passive enhancement of the visual field. This type of fitting has been better received by patients compared to other modalities that created significant image jump or blur induced by the prism gratings.[22] Given that Fresnel prism can be trialed in amounts up to 40 prism diopters or Peli Prism Kits™ (Chadwick Optical) are available close to 60 prism diopters, patients can experience the prism benefits before being fit with a pair of spectacles with permanent placement.[23]

For more detailed information regarding prism placement see the following two sections in this chapter: Understanding Prism Designs for Homonymous Hemianopia and Prism Treatment in Patients with Homonymous Hemianopia. Another option for improving awareness of the missing visual field is to undergo scanning training. By improving saccadic function and developing purposeful eye movements, the individual looks and scans into the missing field and looks for objects in that field.[24] Patients who have long-standing visual field loss often adopt this approach; however, by training efficient scan patterns, patients become more functional with more efficiently.[24]

Both types of approaches to field enhancement benefit from integration of the two techniques with the coordination of care of an orientation and mobility specialist. By addressing not just the field loss but also spatial awareness deficits, patients with field loss improve in their rehabilitation outcomes.

Central Scotomas

Patients with visual impairment often have patterns of vision loss that correlate with their ocular pathology. Macular degeneration, diabetic macular edema or macular holes may cause central blur and central scotomas.[25,26] From mild metamorphopsia through an absolute scotoma, patients need to adapt to their new vision and in severe cases this may require the use of a peripheral retinal point to function.

Patients with central vision loss often mention issues with disabling glare or decreased visual function due to increased lighting.[26] Contrast sensitivity and color vision may be impacted as well.[26] Central scotomas create a challenge for patients as they impede the area of vision that is their normal visual center as well as the area that is responsible for detail vision. This impacts reading small print, facial recognition, and seeing street signs while driving[25]. Amsler grid or microperimetry can be used to measure the central defect.

Depending on the size, location and number of scotomas centrally, patients may have difficulty with the visual resolution of small print. There can also be reduced saccadic efficiency and fixation stability that results in a slower reading speed; approximately 10X slower than someone with normal vision.[25, 27] The size and location of the patient's preferred retinal locus (PRL) may dictate the ability to use their vision for dynamic tasks like reading efficiently and identifying faces. With time, patients typically become more efficient with using their PRL on their own but occasionally may need training.[28]

Depending on the size and severity of a central scotoma, patients have been shown to benefit from Eccentric Viewing (EV) training.[28] This training is geared to help the patient use their PRL more efficiently or to train a new retinal position. EV training often combines the use of fixation and saccadic activities which the patient may do in office but also practice in their home environment. Patients are trained by a rehabilitation professional, such as an occupational therapist or a low vision therapist, over the course of several visits to identify the best peripheral retinal location, and train the patient to utilize this new location, called a trained retinal locus (TRL). Additionally, technology such as microperimeters have training programs that provide biofeedback for patients to learn to use and hold their TRL position.[29]

EV training has been shown to improve reading speeds, increase fixation, and improve visual acuity in some patients but the effect of this may not be long-lasting if the disease process is active. Rubin et al. showed that patients who received EV training did not have an improvement in "task performance, reading performance or fixation stability" compared to controls.[30] In addition, they found that visual acuity worsened, thus demonstrating the progression of the disease process is more significant than the beneficial effects of EV training over the course of the disease.[30]

Treatment options for patients with central scotomas are vast and effective, either individually or in combination with other strategies. Spectacle correction should be assessed to address blur that is the result of uncorrected refractive error.[26] This step in the low vision assessment is also an appropriate time to discuss the benefits and limitations of spectacle correction. Some patients often assume that blur is related to the need for a prescription change when often the blur is the result of ocular pathology.[26] Despite limited acuity improvement, glasses can have additional benefits. Tints can be used to reduce glare complaints and improve contrast; for monocular patients, spectacles with polycarbonate lenses can be used to protect the better seeing eye in case of fall or injury.[31]

Magnification is another option for improving visual function in patients with scotomas. Depending on the patient's visual goal, optical devices such as microscopes or stand magnifiers are effective options to improve visual acuity. For patients who exhibit a range of visual goals or have poor contrast, electronic magnification with video magnification or closed circuit televisions are appropriate. Smart technology such as smart phones and tablets can also be adapted to increase letter size and contrast to help patients maintain their visual goals.

At times, the scotoma a patient experiences may be so large that efficient use of their vision for reading is impossible. An extreme eye or head turn to use their PRL may only offer fleeting fixation stability. In those situations, sight substitution strategies such as audiobooks or tactile strategies: bump dots to give texture to buttons on a microwave can be used. Coordination of in-home training with an occupational therapist or rehabilitation teacher is crucial when implementing these strategies for best effectiveness.

Peripheral Vision Loss

Patients who experience vision loss from glaucoma, retinitis pigmentosa, retinal vascular conditions, and retinal detachment may also report symptoms consistent with CBS.[32] Patients with peripheral vision loss often have difficulty with mobility and may report bumping into objects, walking down stairs or walking uneven surfaces. Patients may also exhibit difficulty with spatial awareness in the form of finding objects on a desk or a book on a shelf.

Depending on the pathology causing their peripheral field loss, patients may also exhibit central vision loss as well as difficulties with contrast sensitivity. Glaucoma is one such condition that causes a multitude of complaints.[33] Observing patients as they walk into the exam room is also incredibly insightful; unfamiliar areas may require the patient to request help or reach out to try to grasp for a railing or trail the wall for orientation. The case history of these patients should include questions about falls or injuries, as well as car accidents or moving violations if the patient is a driver.

For patients with difficulty with orientation of their immediate space, devices for improving visual field are limited. For patients with good visual acuity and contrast sensitivity, a reverse telescope may be an option. This is a device where the patient views through the objective lens of the telescope which minifies the visual field through the telescope.[34] The amount of minification is proportional to the amount of magnification the telescope would provide when used as intended. For example, a telescope that provides 3X magnification will, in turn, produce 3X minification when viewing through the objective lens. Using a field enhancement device can be helpful when the field is extremely reduced but will cause a reduction in contrast and visual acuity, thus impeding the quality of vision through the telescope. This reduction of visual quality may negate the field enhancement properties of the telescope.[34] Trialing these devices are a good option, but expectations should be managed for the patient and the clinician when taking acuity and contrast into consideration.

Reading can also be a challenge for patients who have severe field constriction. Scanning from line to line can be difficult and may only allow a patient to see a word, or even just a few letters at a time. Patients may use their finger or a straight edge to try to keep their place while reading. Optical devices for field expansion in these cases are not often successful due to the impact on visual resolution from the effects of minification. By minifying the letters, visual discrimination may pass the threshold of a patient's ability to see their print.

In situations where reading is impaired due to field of view, magnification strategies will not be useful. Thus, it's best to enhance the remaining acuity with lighting and contrast, while providing maximum acuity for reading. Sometimes despite optimum central acuity, patients may not be able to read at a pace that is commensurate with their needs or desire for reading. In cases where visual reading is not efficient, auditory reading should be considered. Optical character recognition devices can convert printed text to an auditory format, which allows the patient auditory enjoyment of their preferred text. Another option is to use smart technology which may employ apps or accessibility options to read texts or print without needing to search for the beginning line or change contrast options.

Disability Certification

Patients with vision loss may qualify for benefits and services based on their level of visual acuity or field. In the United States, the Social Security Administration governs disability applications and sets limits for qualification for government assistance. This assistance may include tax benefits, application for Medicare, as well as serving as a gateway for state and non-government organizations (NGOs) as a criterion for entry.

The visual acuity requirements were historically based on Snellen projection charts and used 20/200 with best correction in the better-seeing eye as its cutoff acuity for certification. With older projection charts, the levels of acuity jump from 20/100 to 20/200, and thus people whose vision falls between the gap between 20/100 and 20/200 would qualify.[35] To reduce confusion, in 2006 the federal government changed the qualifying acuity to include those optotypes that fell between 20/100 and 20/200 on specialized charts such as the ETDRS Chart or Bailey-Lovie Charts. If the patient cannot see any letter on the 20/100 line with best-corrected vision, they are considered legally blind.[35] Patients are to use their central vision. Testing eccentric viewing positions should not be used with visual acuity testing for disability. Special contact lenses may correct vision beyond the legal blindness cutoff. Sustainable wear must be achieved in order for correction of visual acuity with the contact lens to be used in legal blindness certification.[34]

Visual fields may also be used for legal blindness certification under strict testing conditions. Visual field testing must be tested using a Size III4e isopter and standardized testing. When a central scotoma is significant in size, automated kinetic testing is not allowed, and manual kinetic testing must be performed. To qualify for legal blindness, an individual may have no greater than 20 degrees of field in their widest diameter in their better seeing eye.[35] Appropriate refractive correction must be provided through the use of a trial lens as spectacle frames may impact field of view. While using automated static perimetry, the mean decibel can be used for certification of disability. For mean decibels of –22 decibels or less, patients qualify on 24-2 and 30-2 patterns. For all field measurements, the testing needs to be reliable with good fixation and patient cooperation.

Visual Efficiency Measurement

For patients who do not qualify strictly based on their visual acuity and visual field, a Visual Efficiency Measurement can be used. Visual efficiency uses a combination of both visual acuity and visual field measurements to create a score that describes the patient's overall visual impairment. Percentages are assigned to visual acuities and are listed on the Social Security Website.[35] The visual field component measures the limits of the patient's kinetic visual field on specific meridians (0, 45, 90, 135, 180, 225, 270, and 315) and then divided by 5. The last measurement is the product of the visual acuity efficiency and visual field efficiency. If the product of these two measurements is 20% or less, the patient would qualify as being disabled.

Interprofessional Referrals

Patients with visual decrease may benefit from referrals to rehabilitation professionals. Aspects of daily activities, mobility, and emotional adaptation to vision loss often require further assessment and specialized expertise outside the scope of an ECC.

Referrals to interprofessional and collaborative rehabilitation providers are initiated by the ECC or may be requested by the patient, family members, or support system. Visual acuity and/or field measurements, a formal diagnosis, and rehabilitation goals are required to qualify for some of these resources.

Occupational Therapy

An occupational therapist can work with a patient to address different activities, or occupations, to improve visual function. Occupational therapy is often prescribed by the managing ECC and services may be covered by a patient's medical insurance. Occupational therapists can provide device training, lighting and safety evaluations, adaptive strategies and train on adaptive technologies.[36] For more detailed information regarding occupational therapy, see the Low Vision Rehabilitation section in this chapter.

Certified Orientation and Mobility Specialists (COMS)

Patients with vision loss may have difficulty with independent travel and need to learn skills to allow for safe and confident travel.[36] These specialists are certified in training patients on how to plan routes, learn environmental cues and how to improve their spatial awareness. COMS may train a person on how to use a white cane or teach family members how to be a sighted guide to assist with independent travel. In cases where an individual has mastered their cane skills, they may consider pursuing training with a guide dog.[36] Specialized COMS provide training at guide dog schools and training may take anywhere from one to three months depending on the visually impaired individual's mastery of basic skills.

Driving Rehabilitation Specialists (DRS)

Driving rehabilitation specialists (DRS) provide assessments for fitness to drive, which include cognitive abilities as well as reaction time. DRS can also provide behind-the-wheel training and make suggestions on adaptations to mirrors, steering wheels, and additional modifications depending on the needs of the driver.[36] DRS can also provide training for patients who use bioptic telescopes for driving, and in some states, it is required training for licensure.

Social Workers

Social workers can provide case management, assist with referrals, and provide counseling to patients with visual impairments. Social workers assist with transportation resources, counseling, coordinating support groups for patients and family members, and patient advocacy. They also provide psychosocial assessments and help patients and family members adjust to difficulties and challenges that arise from adapting to vision loss.[36]

Patients who experience vision loss require a multidisciplinary approach to addressing not just the visual changes, but also the impact of these changes on everyday function. When working with individuals with vision loss, it is important to consider referrals to these rehabilitation professionals to manage any noted difficulties.[36]

—Karen Squier

Understanding Prism Designs for Homonymous Hemianopia

Introduction

Homonymous Hemianopia (HH) is a debilitating condition that often results from an intracranial stroke. Two of the most frequent quality-of-life concerns of individuals with HH are driving and mobility. Assessing a patient's ability to successfully drive is one that should be considered in tandem with your state/country's legislative visual field requirements. Eyeglasses are a potentially powerful tool to help patients maximize the utility of a patient's remaining vision. This section will review various types of eyeglass lens designs, and how they interact with a patient's visual system.

Principles of Homonymous Hemianopia

There are some critical principles to keep in mind when working with an HH patient:

1. A patient being cognizant and aware that they are afflicted with HH does not mean that they are constantly cognitively aware of the implications of their condition and their missing visual field. While you may be able to design exercises and games that allow them to enhance detection and awareness in a controlled environment, how these skills translate to function in an uncontrolled environment is unclear. Ultimately, our goal is to help the patient navigate uncontrolled environments.

2. Peripheral vision works by detecting motion and providing a cue to direct your gaze. Gaze shifts and head movements are heavily influenced by what is detected in the peripheral vision. The HH patient is missing those cues, and their eye movements are influenced accordingly.

3. Eyeglasses are essentially a static device being placed over a dynamic system of eye movements. You must consider the implications of how the eyes, and

the visual field will interact with the eyeglasses in various circumstances that you may not normally be prone to consider.

4. The patient's visual field is constantly interacting with the eyeglasses. It's important to verify and consider the patient's entire visual field.

When designing lenses to interact and expand awareness for a patient with HH, we are often utilizing high-powered prisms and interacting with the visual system in a somewhat novel fashion. As we explore this novelty, it's important to differentiate the forms and sensitivity of what we generically refer to as "double vision." Functionally, the eyes are only bothered by double vision when it occurs along the horopter. Other than that small focal area, the eyes are in a constant state of double vision. While we don't want to interfere with the sensitive form of double vision, we can utilize the insensitive form to enhance awareness in the blind area.

When using high-powered prisms, it's also important to remember that when a prism redirects light, it redirects it from somewhere else. The place from which it's redirecting light is no longer visible and creates a gap in the vision. The gap that is created by the prism in the patient's visual field is referred to as an apical scotoma. While mounting high-powered prisms in glasses, we can mitigate the discomfort caused by an apical scotoma by locating it outside the horopter.

To further elaborate on the concept of apical scotoma, consider a round bifocal. When a patient directs their gaze into a +3.00 diopter add of a round bifocal, they experience an image jump of approximately 3.3 prism diopters. This translates to roughly 1.6 degrees of apical scotoma. The prisms used in hemianopia lens design are much stronger than this—between 10 and 65 prism diopters, which would create an apical scotoma covering between 5 and 35 degrees of visual field. We will discuss the implications of this effect as we review the various lens designs. A thorough detailed review of the various prism options and how they function, accompanied by extensive figure illustrations are available as an online resource in the Ancillary material section of Chapter 9.

—Charlie Saccarelli

Prism Treatment in Patients with Homonymous Hemianopia

Introduction

In patients with homonymous hemianopia, prism can be used to expand what remains of the functional visual field by shifting images from areas of visual loss into areas of intact vision.

Prescribing Prism

Prism can be incorporated throughout both lenses (yoked prism) or put only in a portion of the lenses. The greatest treatment success has been found using prism placed above and below the visual axis. Here, the prism is placed monocularly on the lens corresponding to the side of the hemianopia with the base oriented toward the side of the hemianopia. Forty prism diopter segments on the upper and lower parts of the lens provide 20 degrees of visual field expansion.[37] One can obtain up to 30 degrees of field expansion with 57 prism diopter prisms.[38]

Obliquely oriented prism allows expansion of the central visual field. Because the image still falls on peripheral retina, the patient does not experience double vision. Here, two prism segments are placed 11 mm apart, above and below the line of sight, unilaterally on the lens corresponding to the side of the hemianopia. The upper prism is placed with the base out and down at a 30 degrees angle from the horizontal. The lower prism is placed with the base out and up at an angle of 30 degrees from the horizontal. Treatment with either horizontal or oblique prism can be accomplished with ground-in prism or temporary stick-on prisms.

Multiperiscopic prisms involve a device with 3–4 half-penta prisms that shift the image the equivalent of 100 prism diopters. The device is placed on the front of one lens, above and below the line of sight, with the base 20 degrees relative to horizontal. This provides approximately 42 degrees of lateral field expansion.[39] This compares to an obliquely oriented Fresnel prism of 65 prism diopters that provides 32 degrees of field expansion.[39]

Prism Training and Adaptation

Training in the use of field-expanding prism is critical. Patients look through the central portion of the glasses and move their eyes normally. They should not look through the prism, as this will result in diplopia. Once they detect an object in the peripheral vision, they turn their head to fixate on the object through the prism-free center of the lens.

Monocular prism segments can improve quality of life, improve mobility, and allow avoidance of obstacles.[20, 39, 40] Between 41% and 70% of patients continue to use the prism glasses long term.[38, 41] Drivers using oblique prism of 40 prism diopters have improved the ability to recognize unexpected hazards compared to those with sham prism.[42] Likewise, obliquely placed prism of 57 prism diopters improves the ability to detect objects on the blind side and expands the visual field of those with complete hemianopia up to 115 degrees.[20, 41, 43] This field expansion would allow one to legally drive in some states.

Unfortunately, there are downsides to using prism to expand the visual field. Field expansion with prism is aimed at expanding the visual field in the distance. Because the prism is within the area of fixation when looking down, patients will experience double vision when looking down to read. A separate pair of reading glasses is necessary to avoid this. Similarly, patients may have trouble going down stairs as they look downward through the prism. Other challenges associated with the use of prism to expand the visual field include being startled by objects jumping into the field of vision and the optical quality of the temporary stick-on prisms. Permanent, ground-in prism should be used if long-term wear is desired.

—Denise Goodwin

Low Vision Rehabilitation

Introduction

Occupational therapy is a valuable component of treatment for CBS in helping individuals improve independence in their daily life. The American Occupational Therapy Association defines occupational therapy as "the therapeutic use of everyday life occupations with persons, groups, or populations [i.e., clients] to support occupational performance and participation."[44] People with disabilities or injuries often face obstacles that affect their independence and ability to complete daily activities. These everyday engagements are referred to in occupational therapy as "occupations." Occupations are personally meaningful and goal-directed pursuits that people need, want, or are expected to do. They are composed of activities—more general actions—and tasks, which are the smallest units of action. For example, the occupation of preparing a meal may include the activity of cooking, which involves tasks such as chopping vegetables or boiling water. Common occupations include dressing, grocery shopping, socializing, reading, driving, and engaging in leisure. An occupational therapist's goal is to improve an individual's independence with these meaningful activities.

Role of Occupational Therapy

Occupational therapy practitioners (OTPs) play a critical role in supporting individuals with CBS. Low vision rehabilitation focuses on enhancing independence by using targeted strategies and skills tailored to the patient's visual impairment. Comprehensive assessment and personalized treatment planning involves evaluating how visual hallucinations impact daily functioning, identifying environmental triggers that contribute to visual hallucinations, and addressing barriers to occupational engagement such as reduced social participation. Through the development of an occupational profile, OTPs integrate client-specific factors and contextual influences to adequately guide interventions that enhance an individual's independence, promote adaptive strategies, provide targeted education, and support overall well-being in the presence of visual impairment.

Evaluation

Low vision occupational therapists conduct comprehensive evaluations to assess an individual's functional independence in daily activities by evaluating how generalized visual impairments affect occupational performance and determining the level of assistance required to complete daily occupations (Figure 9.22). The impact and factors that may contribute to CBS visual hallucination frequency are explored. The patient's current understanding of their condition, and the amount of education, resources, or referrals that may be needed are also evaluated. Visual hallucinations may affect the patient's ability to ambulate safely and navigate fall hazards. A home lighting assessment promotes safer ambulation or improved performance with desired occupations.[45] If poor lighting is a contributing factor for the patient experiencing CBS, addressing this may aid in the decrease of hallucinations.[46] Low vision and CBS are linked to

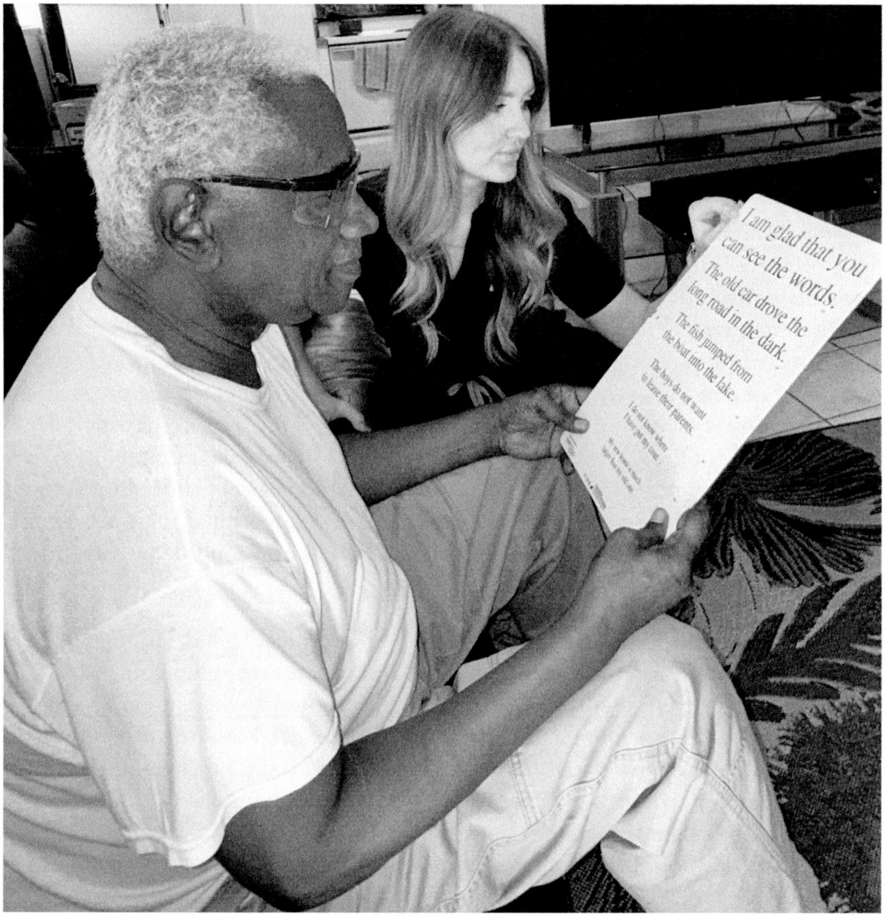

Figure 9.22 A patient sits on a couch with yellow tinted lenses while an occupational therapist assesses critical print size.

psychosocial challenges in older adults, so social participation and isolation risk are assessed.[47] Optical devices, assistive technology, and appropriate visual skills are needed to improve functional vision. Improving functional vision can often reduce the frequency or intensity of visual hallucinations associated with CBS.[48] By the conclusion of an evaluation, an OTP synthesizes information gathered from objective assessments, subjective reports, and clinical observations to create a client-centered plan of care. The plan targets the individual's goals and often includes rehabilitation training, environmental modifications, and adaptive strategies to support meaningful engagement in daily life.

Intervention

Intervention strategies that incorporate behavioral techniques, environmental modification, applying adaptive technology or utilizing distraction may help

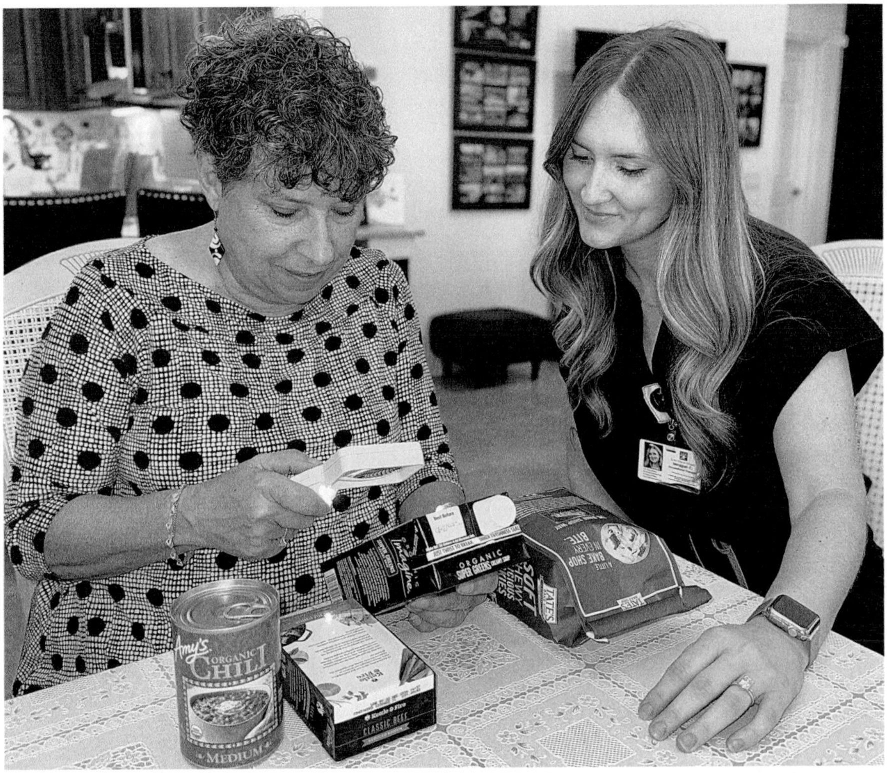

Figure 9.23 A patient seated at a table with an occupational therapist using a handheld magnifier to read food labels.

manage visual hallucinations. Use is made of visual techniques, including eye movement exercises such as rapid blinking, directed ocular movements, and focusing directly at the hallucinations. Sleep is a vital occupation essential for overall well-being, so stress management and sleep quality through the implementation of sleep hygiene habits such as routine strategies and relaxation techniques should also be addressed.

Adaptive technology and assistive devices—such as magnifiers, electronic magnification systems, or low vision optical aids and tools that are prescribed by an eye doctor—help maximize the patient's remaining vision. Research indicates that using the patient's remaining vision often decreases the frequency of visual hallucinations.[47] Using tools such as handheld magnifiers to read food labels, electronic magnification for prescription instructions, and specialized glasses for meal preparations, while providing personalized instruction on how to integrate custom low vision glasses in functional scenarios, enhances independence in daily routines (Figure 9.23).

Although CBS is not a cognitive disorder, it can significantly affect psychosocial aspects of a patient's life. OTPs identify meaningful, client-centered

Table 9.2 Patient goals and corresponding interventions

Patient goals and corresponding interventions	
Patient goal	**Intervention examples**
• Prepare a meal independently	• Introduce adaptive kitchen utensils, promote high contrast, teach safety techniques, utilize tactile and audio labels, improve lighting
• Navigate Familiar and Unfamiliar Environments Safely	• Improve lighting, assess home environment (i.e. clear pathways), add high contrast tape to stairs, encourage use of mobility aids, education on management of visual hallucinations affecting safe ambulation
• Read Food Labels, Prescriptions, Menus	• Utilize optical aids such as magnifiers, improve task lighting, teach effective low vision reading techniques
• Participate in Social Settings	• Teach self-advocacy skills, education on transportation options, encourage attending support groups
• Engage in Leisure Activities	• Adapt activities as needed, encourage utilization of optical and assistive devices, educate on glare management if needed

activities—such as participating in low vision support groups, engaging in adapted community events, or resuming valued hobbies with environmental modifications—and integrate these into individualized treatment plans to enhance social participation and emotional well-being for individuals with low vision and CBS. Strategies such as cognitive restructuring—identifying and adapting unhelpful thinking that may lead to emotional distress—can help patients manage symptoms and improve social participation.[49] Other strategic and supportive interventions include collaborative goal setting to reduce fear-driven isolation and enhancing a patient's daily functioning.[50, 51] Goal setting is an important component of cognitive-behavioral frame of reference (Table 9.2). Implementation allows the patient and therapist team to create measurable and attainable goals in relation to the management of visual hallucinations. OTPs also utilize role play and muscle relaxation, allowing patients to practice various management strategies for effective use during their visual hallucinations.

Education and Collaboration

Among the most beneficial first steps in assisting a patient with CBS are providing comprehensive education to the patient, caregiver, and family.[52] This often alleviates distress associated with visual hallucinations. Often, patients with CBS have trouble articulating symptoms or feelings to caregivers and family members. Informed inquiry to explore the patient's lived experience and any communication barriers ensures all individuals involved in the care process are equipped to understand the condition and fulfill any supportive role effectively.

OTPs can connect patients with local resources, educate on community programs, and teach advocacy skills.[53, 54] Limited public awareness of CBS makes it more difficult for individuals to find others who understand their symptoms.[47, 55] A close collaboration between patients and OTPs enables identifying additional needs and necessary referrals to other appropriate professionals—such as physical therapists, orientation and mobility specialists, rehabilitation counselors, or mental health professionals—ensuring comprehensive individualized care.

Conclusion

OTPs with specialty training in low vision provide comprehensive evaluations and individualized treatments assisting CBS patients in maximizing their remaining vision and improving independence. Utilizing occupational interventions allows patients to adapt to daily life with visual hallucinations. These interventions include personalized training in the use of assistive devices, adapting environments, providing patient education, addressing social participation, and demonstrating the use of compensatory techniques. The goal is to allow those with low vision and CBS to maintain their independence, participation in meaningful occupations, and overall well-being.

Additional low vision rehabilitation figures 9.4–9.21 are available as an online resource in the Ancillary material section of Chapter 9.

—Meagan Chapman

REFERENCES

1. Ord LM et al., Looking at Charles Bonnet syndrome: Prevalence and experiences of patients attending a vision rehabilitation clinic. *J Vis Impair Blindness*. 2018;112(5):488–96.
2. Jones L et al., *Arch Dis Child*. 2025. doi:10.1136/archdischild-2024-327811
3. Chai YX et al., *Br J Ophthalmol*. 2023;107(3):361–6. doi:10.1136/bjophthalmol-2021-319655
4. Rahmati M et al., *PLoS One*. 2025. doi:10.1371/journal.pone.0317452
5. Gothwal VK et al., *Ophthalmic Physiol Opt*. 2023. doi:10.1111/opo.13055
6. Dougherty BE et al., *Optom Vis Sci*. 2011. doi:10.1097/OPX.0b013e31822a61e7
7. Seiple W et al., *Transl Vis Sci Technol*. 2025. doi:10.1167/tvst.14.1.3
8. Vukicevic M et al., *Clin Exp Ophthalmol*. 2008. doi:10.1111/j.1442-9071.2008.01814.x

9. Okudo AC et al., A comparative analysis of anxiety and depression among glaucoma and cataractous patients in southwest Nigeria. *Open J Ophthalmol.* 2021;11(2).
10. Court H et al., *BMC Med.* 2014. doi:10.1186/s12916-014-0181-7
11. Dillon L et al., *Eye (Lond).* 2020. doi:10.1038/s41433-020-0992-z
12. Adair DK et al., *Am J Psychiatry.* 1988. doi:10.1176/ajp.145.7.895b
13. Niazi S et al., *Acta Ophthalmol.* 2020. doi:10.1111/aos.14287. PMID: 31654492
14. White UE et al., *Transl Vis Sci Technol.* 2022. doi:10.1167/tvst.11.1.34
15. Thayaparan K et al., *Br J Ophthalmol.* 2006. doi:10.1136/bjo.2006.109280
16. Ffytche DH, *Dialogues Clin Neurosci.* 2007. doi:10.31887/DCNS.2007.9.2/dffytche
17. Pang L, *Optom Vis Sci.* 2016. doi:10.1097/OPX.0000000000000959
18. Hartney KE et al., *J Psychiatr Pract.* 2011. doi:10.1097/01.pra.0000396067.87343.fb
19. Peli E et al., *Optom Vis Sci.* 2017. doi:10.1097/OPX.0000000000001102
20. Goodwin D, *Clin Ophthalmol.* 2014. doi:10.2147/OPTH.S59452
21. Sand KM et al., *Acta Neurol Scand Suppl.* 2013. doi:10.1111/ane.12050
22. Peli E et al., *Optom Vis Sci.* 2016. doi:10.1097/OPX.0000000000000820
23. Chadwick Optical, https://chadwickoptical.com/products/the-peli-lens/ [cited July 6, 2025]
24. Bouwmeester L et al., *J Neurol Neurosurg Psychiatry.* 2007. doi:10.1136/jnnp.2006.103853
25. Silvestri V et al., *Ophthalmic Physiol Opt.* 2020. doi:10.1111/opo.12726
26. Sunness JS et al., *Ophthalmology.* 2010. doi:10.1016/j.ophtha.2009.11.017
27. Chung STL, *Ophthalmic Physiol Opt.* 2020. doi:10.1111/opo.12664
28. Chung STL, Training to improve speed of letter recognition benefits reading speed in people with central vision loss. *Invest Ophthalmol Vis Sci.* 2018;59:630
29. Lewerenz D et al., *Clin Exp Optom.* 2018. doi:10.1111/cxo.12602
30. Rubin GS et al., Eccentric viewing training for age-related macular disease: Results of a randomized controlled trial (the EFFECT Study). *Ophthalmol Sci.* 2023;4(2):100422
31. Bailie M et al., *Clin Exp Optom.* 2013. doi:10.1111/cxo.12031
32. Lomo T et al., *Acta Ophthalmol.* 2021. doi:10.1111/aos.14620
33. Kaleem MA et al., *Ophthalmol Glaucoma.* 2019. doi:10.1016/j.ogla.2019.01.012
34. Brilliant RL et al., Rehabilitation of peripheral visual field defects. In: Brilliant RL, ed, *Essentials of Low Vision Practice.* Boston: Butterworth Heinemann; 1999:251–65
35. Disability Evaluation Under Social Security 2.00 Special Senses and Speech - Adult. https://www.ssa.gov/disability/professionals/bluebook/2.00-SpecialSensesandSpeech-Adult.htm [cited July 8, 2025]

36. Vision Professionals, AER. https://aerbvi.memberclicks.net/visionprofessionals, retrieved 5/5/2025
37. Bowers AR et al., Community-based trial of a peripheral prism visual field expansion device for hemianopia. *Arch Ophthalmol.* 2008;126:657–64
38. Bowers AR et al., Randomized crossover clinical trial of real and sham peripheral prism glasses for hemianopia. *JAMA Ophthalmol.* 2014;132:214–22
39. Bowers AR et al., Pilot study of a pedestrian collision detection test for a multisite trial of field expansion devices for hemianopia. *Optom Vis Sci.* 2024;101:408–16
40. O'Neill EC et al., Prism therapy and visual rehabilitation in homonymous visual field loss. *Optom Vis Sci.* 2011;88:263–8
41. Houston KE et al., Driving with hemianopia VI: Peripheral prisms and perceptual-motor training improve detection in a driving simulator. *Transl Vis Sci Technol.* 2018;7:5
42. Bowers AR et al., A pilot evaluation of on-road detection performance by drivers with hemianopia using oblique peripheral prisms. *Stroke Res Treat.* 2012;2012:176806
43. Moss AM et al., Patients with homonymous hemianopia become visually qualified to drive using novel monocular sector prisms. *J Neuroophthalmol.* 2014;34:53–6
44. Occupational therapy practice framework: Domain and process, 4th edn. *Am J Occupat Ther* [Internet]. 2020;74(Suppl_2). Available from: www.research.aota.org/ajot doi:10.5014/ajot.2020.74s2001 [cited April 15, 2025]
45. Øien TB, *Front Rehabil Sci.* 2022. doi:10.3389/fresc.2022.829903
46. Pang L, *Optom Vis Sci.* 2016. doi:10.1097/OPX.0000000000000959
47. Fraser S et al., *BMJ Open.* 2019. doi:10.1136/bmjopen-2019-029940
48. Singh A et al., Charles Bonnet syndrome improves when treatment is effective in age-related macular degeneration. *Br J Ophthalmol.* 2010;95(2):291–2
49. Slepecky M, *Eur Psych.* 2017. doi:10.26226/morressier.5885d714d462b8028d8917db
50. Guttman et al., Adaptations for low vision [Internet]. 2022. Available from: https://www.escrs.org/eurotimes/adaptations-for-low-vision [cited May 19, 2025]
51. Kaldenberg J et al., Occupational therapy practice guidelines for older adults with low vision. *Am J Occupat Ther* [Internet]. 2020;74(2). Available from: https://research.aota.org/ajot/article-abstract/74/2/7402397010p1/9869/Occupational-Therapy-Practice-Guidelines-for-Older?redirectedFrom=fulltext doi:10.5014/ajot.2020.742003 [cited April 5, 2025]
52. Vandendooren M et al., *The Theory and Practice of Low Vision Rehabilitation* [training material]. Sarasota, FL: Low Vision Works; 2020
53. Scheiman M et al., *Low Vision Rehabilitation: A Practical Guide for Occupational Therapists.* Thorofare, NJ: Slack Incorp; 2003:11–4

54. Whittaker S et al., *Low Vision Rehabilitation: A Practical Guide for Occupational Therapists*. New York, NY: Routledge; 2024:136–7
55. Ord LM et al., *J Vis Impair Blind* [Internet]. 2018. https://journals.sagepub.com/doi/abs/10.1177/0145482X1811200506 doi:10.1177/0145482x1811200506

Chapter 10

ILLUSTRATIVE PATIENT CASE REPORTS

Leonid Skorin, Jr., Andrew Krein, Donald Morris, Emily Stiles, James Hall, Anmol Gosai, Jeffrey Holt, Jasmyne Jenkins, John F. Renfro and Gary M. Cusick

Introduction

"No bubble is so iridescent or floats longer than that blown by the successful teacher."[1]

—Sir William Osler

There are a wide variety of pathological processes, both ocular and intracranial, that can cause significant vision loss, resulting in a patient having visual hallucinations that form the basis of Charles Bonnet Syndrome (CBS). In addition, CBS itself may have a myriad of ways it can present and have an innumerable number of visual hallucinations that patients may perceive. For clinical entities such as CBS, well-written and narrative patient case reports are still a great learning tool. This chapter presents a number of patient case reports written by many different practitioners. It details their CBS patients and, most importantly, how they addressed the patients' concerns. Each clinician explains how they approached helping the patient and their caregivers better understand and successfully navigate this syndrome. As Dr. William Osler's epigram states, hopefully each of these patient case reports acts as a bubble of knowledge that assists the reader in helping with their own CBS patients.

—Leonid Skorin, Jr.

Case 1

A 100-year-old female presented to the eye clinic with complaints of recent-onset visual hallucinations. She claimed she saw three young children, including a smaller boy who was persistently hopping up and down, next to two girls who were stationary. She described them as well-dressed and looking "cute." Occasionally, she would see a fourth child. She quickly realized that this fourth child was actually herself from her youth. She knew these images were not real. She also stated she was unafraid of these images and believed that the children were there to "protect" her and watch over her.

The patient's previous ocular history included end-stage glaucoma in both eyes. She used timolol 0.5% two times daily and latanoprost 0.005% at bedtime in

DOI: 10.1201/9781003633365-10

both eyes as treatment. She had selective laser trabeculoplasty in both eyes in the past. One year ago, her visual acuity was 20/80 right eye and 20/400 left eye. However, on today's visual acuity reading, she could only recognize hand motion when looking out of the right eye and 20/500 when looking out of the left eye. There is no reported history of psychiatric illness or of hearing voices. Additionally, the patient was oriented to time, place, and person.

Her intraocular pressure was recorded at 15mmHg right eye and 16mmHg left eye. The patient's slit-lamp exam was unremarkable, and she was pseudophakic in both eyes. Both optic nerves showed cup-to-disc ratios of 0.9. The fundus in the left eye was unremarkable except for macular mottling and a few small scattered drusen. The right eye fundus showed the typical "blood and thunder," as seen in a central retinal vein occlusion (CRVO) (Figure 10.1). There also appeared to be significant hemorrhages and edema in the macula (Figure 10.1).

The sudden drop in visual acuity, especially in the right eye from the CRVO, most probably resulted in the patient experiencing these visual hallucinations. This patient's hallucinations are unique since she exhibited a combination of both static (two stationary girls) and dynamic (boy who was constantly hopping up and down in a repetitive and stereotypical fashion) imagery in addition to exhibiting autoscopy (seeing an image of herself as a young child). The patient was reassured that the images resulted from the further deterioration in the vision in both her eyes. The patient was actually pleased to know that her visual hallucinations had a medical term, Charles Bonnet Syndrome, and that there was a possibility that as her retinal hemorrhages resolved in the right eye,

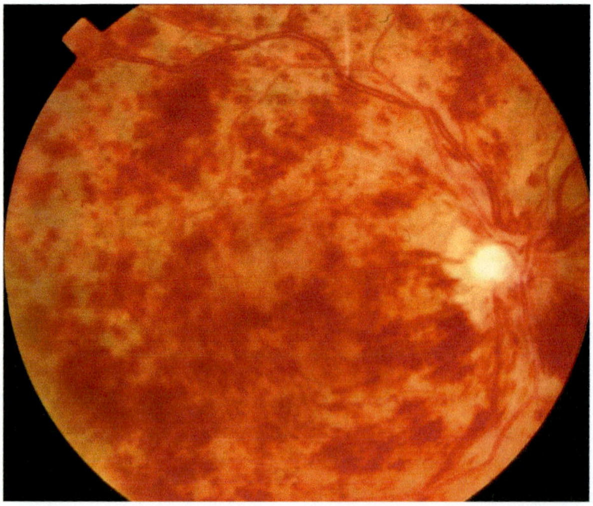

Figure 10.1 Central retinal vein occlusion with macular edema, right eye. With permission, Zaman M, Skorin L, The ophthalmologist's map to Charles Bonnet Syndrome. (2023) Eyes On Eyecare. https://eyesoneyecare.com/resources/ophthalmologists-map-to-charles-bonnet-syndrome/.

the visual hallucinations may disappear. An appointment was scheduled with an internist for an evaluation of a possible systemic etiology for her CRVO. She was also scheduled with a retina specialist for evaluation and possible intervention for the macular edema.

Case submitted by Leonid Skorin, Jr., DO, OD, MS, FAAO, FAOCO, Mayo Clinic Health System, Albert Lea, MN, USA.

Case 2

A 98-year-old Caucasian female presented for a routine eye examination with a chief complaint that her reading was very challenging. This patient was new to the clinic and came with a good recollection of her ocular history. She stated that she had uncomplicated cataract surgery in both eyes performed over twenty years ago and that she also has active neovascular macular degeneration. The patient is actively receiving anti-VEGF (vascular endothelial growth factor) injections every six weeks in her right eye. She did not have any history of cognitive decline, psychiatric disorders, or other systemic conditions that could lead to visual hallucinations. She was fully oriented to time, place, and person during the examination.

On examination, her visual acuity in the right eye (OD) was 20/400. In her left eye (OS), her vision was hand motion (HM). Intraocular pressure was measured at OD: 12 mmHg and OS: 12 mmHg using Goldmann applanation tonometry. The patient was pseudophakic in both eyes, and the cup-to-disc ratio was OD: 0.4 and OS: 0.4. Funduscopic examination showed significant macular disruptions in both eyes, worse in the OS, consistent with advanced macular degeneration. The fundus showed a large area of pale hypopigmented zones in the central macular region of both eyes with adjacent drusen bodies in the area. The size of the atrophic region in the OS was larger than the OD. Optical coherence tomography (OCT) imaging revealed very pronounced macular disruption in both eyes. The OD showed a choroidal neovascular membrane, while OS had a large area of geographic atrophy (Figures 10.2 a, b). The patient's refraction was unchanged, but the patient appeared to benefit from additional high-add powered reading spectacles.

After the exam, I began a line of questioning that allowed for Charles Bonnet-like symptoms to be broached. At first, the patient was hesitant but she then began to explain various visual hallucinations in which she has experienced for the past four years. She reports that these hallucinations are transient in length, but consistent in timing. She states that when she sits in the lunchroom of her senior care home, she is always greeted with an old lady, whom she has never met, seated across the table from her. She reports that as soon as they lock eyes the lady across the table winks at her, and then her hair begins to grow. The patient states that the hair grows to the length of the floor, and when it cannot grow any further, "poof…it all falls out." Furthermore, after this lady's hair falls out, she also disappears. At this time, the patient can then enjoy their lunch. The patient reports that this specific hallucination has been ongoing for the last eight months, with no increase in frequency. After each of these visual hallucinations,

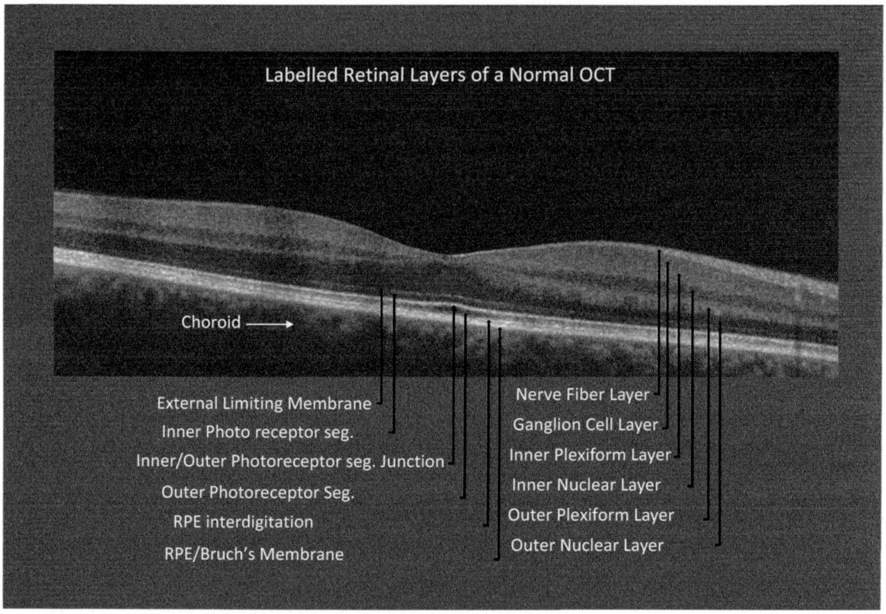

(a)

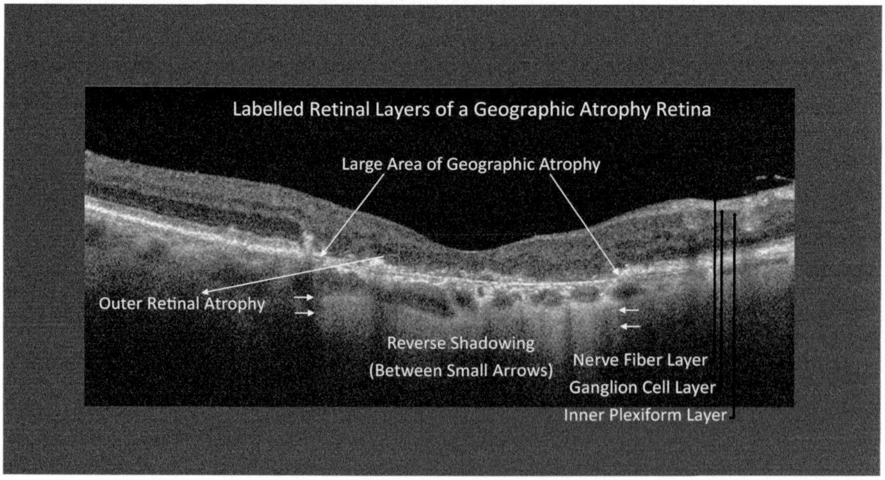

(b)

Figure 10.2 (a) Zeiss Cirrus 500 SD-OCT scan over the fovea in a patient with normal retinal anatomy. This patient has good foveal contour, well-opposed retinal layers and a healthy choroidal appearance. The Retinal Pigment Epithelium (RPE) is well formed and void of any early signs of macular disruption. (b) Zeiss Cirrus 500 SD-OCT scan over the fovea in a patient with advanced age-related macular degeneration with geographic atrophy. In this image there is outer retinal atrophy which the damage includes a host of different structures such as the retinal pigment epithelium, inner segment/outer segment (IS/OS) junction, cone outer segments, external limiting membrane (ELM), and the outer nuclear layer. The Bruch's membrane and choroidal capillaris is visible due to the overlying outer retinal atrophy which leads to signal bleed-through deeper into the choroid called reverse shadowing.

the patient reports she would go back to her room and perform some level of introspection, which, in some instances, would occupy the remainder of her day. She stated that she knew she was never scared of this woman, dually knowing that she was not indeed real but a visual hallucination since her other table mates at lunch never saw this woman. The patient stated that she was concerned for her mental wellbeing during this time.

The doctor took time to explain Charles Bonnet Syndrome (CBS) to the patient, reassuring her that what she was seeing was indeed a visual hallucination and not mental decline. This patient was extremely grateful for an explanation and felt immense relief knowing she was experiencing something related to her vision and not her mental capacity. She divulged there was a certain level of resentment to previous providers for never educating her about the potential for visual disturbances. On a one-year follow-up examination, this patient reported that her mental wellbeing has increased since the phenomena of CBS was explained to her. She spends less time thinking about these visual hallucinations and questioning herself. She currently is aware that she is mentally fit and reports thinking the visual hallucinations are now funny.

I took this opportunity to educate her primary care doctor and the retinal specialist of her CBS. There was a referral to the Institute of the Blind to offer low-vision aids to help with her reading. The patient now uses a handheld tablet magnifier to read her books and is very happy.

Case Submitted by: Andrew Krein, OD, BSc., Devon Eye Clinic, Devon, AB, Canada.

Case 3

The patient first presented to my office when she was in her mid-80s. At that time, she had significant cataracts and macular degeneration (AMD). She left our practice for about six years and while away had cataract surgery on the right eye. When she returned, she had been diagnosed with Charles Bonnet Syndrome (CBS) by an outside doctor. Her symptoms were mainly those of seeing spots and floaters in both eyes. These spots and floaters would either overlap the background or compose the background of whatever she was looking at. Interestingly, these spots had occurred prior to her cataract surgery and resolved after she had cataract surgery and intravitreal injections for the exudative AMD in her right eye.

She eventually returned to my practice in April of 2017 at the age of 91. At that time, she was not experiencing any visual hallucinations. Her vision would vary between 20/50 and 20/60 in her right eye and count finger (CF) vision in her left eye. She was receiving intravitreal injections from a retina specialist for her exudative AMD of the right eye. She also had a large macular scar from previously treated exudative AMD in her left eye. Her intraocular pressure was 17mmHg both eyes and the cup-to-disc ratio was 0.4 both eyes.

She complained about dimming and loss of peripheral vision in her left eye, so she underwent cataract surgery on the left eye in June of 2018. She regained brightness and improved peripheral vision in her left eye.

In March of 2019, the patient noticed white spots in the vision of both her eyes. Her vision at that time was 20/50 in her right eye and CF in her left eye. She stated that her CBS had resurfaced. She was aware that it was CBS, and she was bothered by this. She was counseled that these are visual hallucinations, and that they had nothing to do with her mental status. I explained to her that it does have to do with her brain trying to create visual stimulation. She accepted that but was still bothered by these visual hallucinations.

In June of 2019, the patient's daughter called to state that her mother was seeing more spots and now having other visual hallucinations. I explained again that this was indeed the CBS continuing to manifest itself and that there was nothing we can treat regarding the visual hallucinations. I emphasized that these visual hallucinations do not signify dementia or other mental status conditions. The patient and her family wanted to know if there was a specialist they could see. I did offer an appointment with a neuro-ophthalmologist, but the patient declined.

Over the course of the next few months, the patient would come to the office for recurrent corneal erosion issues. Each time she would say that her visual hallucinations were worsening. Initially, these visual hallucinations manifested only as dots. Then she said, " It was just flowers or circles but I'm now seeing people not just flowers". This was in August of 2019. The visual hallucinations of people really bothered her, even though she understood that this was not due to dementia or mental status issues. Her vision continued to decline in the right eye from the AMD. She was now 20/100 in the right eye and CF in the left eye.

In February of 2020, her vision remained 20/100 right eye and CF left eye. She complained about an increase in the visual hallucinations. This bothered her enough that she was prescribed Risperdal (risperidone) by her psychiatrist; this is an atypical antipsychotic, which she ultimately did not take.

Six months later, in August of 2020, her vision dropped to 20/400 in her right eye and remained CF in the left eye. At one of her eye examinations, she stated she has had "CBS for 10+ years" and "it's still there every day." She did have a period of it going away after her right eye cataract surgery.

In February of 2021, she returned because now she was seeing silver flashes in her left eye. She had continued to be aware of the dark spot in the center of her vision of her left eye from her AMD which appeared unchanged, but these silver flashes were a new symptom. A complete eye examination did not reveal any new ocular pathology, and these silver flashes did go away over time. Interestingly, at this exam, she mentioned that she had not seen any visual hallucinations for a period of time after her eye exam, six months ago. She expressed pleasure that the visual hallucinations had gone away.

Her visual hallucinations of silver flashing lights did again return shortly after the eye exam. I saw the patient at six-monthly intervals from 2021, until she passed away in 2025. Her vision dropped to hand motion in both eyes secondary to her deteriorating AMD. In exams after her second brief respite from the hallucinations, she would complain off and on about seeing things that aren't there, and she was still disturbed that she was seeing people. I would reinforce each time that these were not a mental issue, though unfortunately that did not seem to give her much comfort.

This was a case of CBS with varied and increasing visual hallucinations secondary to vision loss first from cataracts and AMD, then from worsening AMD. There were also two periods when the visual hallucinations were resolved for a short interval. In this case, the patient understood, and accepted, that the hallucinations were not from any mental status issues, but they still bothered her significantly anyway. It was the visual hallucinations of people that especially appeared to bother her.

Case submitted by Donald Morris, DO, FAOCO, South Hills Eye Associates, Pittsburgh, PA, USA.

Case 4

A 94-year-old Caucasian female presented to the eye clinic with a complaint of recent-onset visual hallucinations. She was seeing people crossing the road while riding in the car that her daughter was driving. Her daughter did not see these same people. The patient was concerned that her daughter was going to hit these "pedestrians." The daughter explained that her mother's hallucination recurred many times, and no such "pedestrians" were ever present on the road. Besides the "pedestrians," the patient also saw a forest of trees whenever she was in her daughter's car; similarly, in her home, she would see a cat even though she did not own one.

The patient had previously complained of a purple splash in her vision that gave her surroundings a purplish hue. This purplish vision would last for a few hours and then fade. The patient also complained of severe eye pain, that she thought was the result of her accompanying neck pain.

The patient's past ocular history was significant for multiple branch retinal artery occlusions in both eyes. She also had moderate non-exudative (dry) macular degeneration (AMD), as seen on optical coherence tomography (Figures 10.4 a, b), and advanced glaucoma in both eyes. Her visual acuity was counting fingers right eye and hand motion left eye. Her intraocular pressure was 11mmHg right eye and 12mmHg left eye. An evaluation for arteritic ischemic optic neuropathy (temporal arteritis) was negative and her other systemic stroke workups after finding the occlusion were also negative. Her ophthalmic medications include cyclosporine both eyes as needed for dry eyes and netarsudil 0.02% nightly for glaucoma. She does not receive any treatment for her macular degeneration, nor does she take any oral nutraceuticals. The patient has no other significant medical or psychiatric history.

Her visual symptoms come from three independent issues that can lead to the diagnosis of Charles Bonnet Syndrome (CBS). Her history of continuous branch retinal artery occlusions seems to be the main culprit, combined with her history

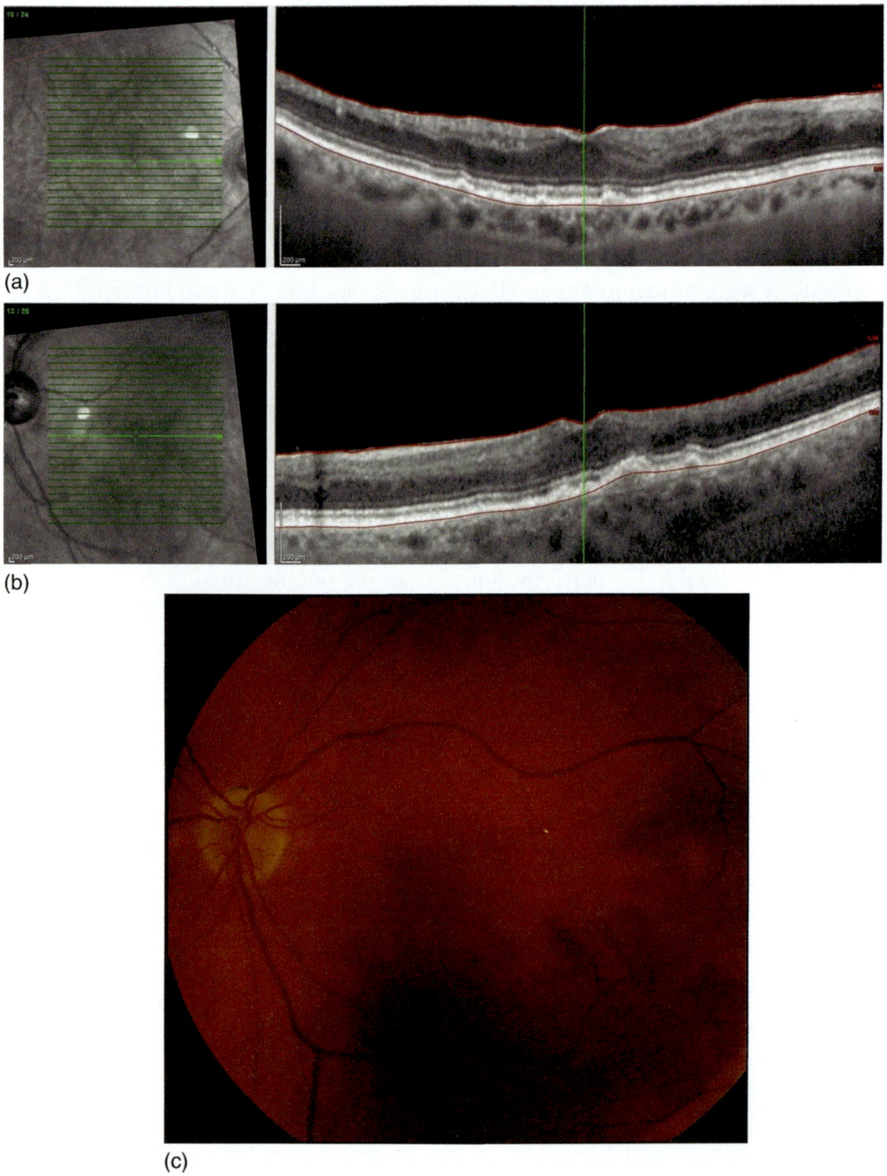

Figure 10.4 (a) Optical coherence tomography of macula right eye: Thinning consistent with nerve fiber layer loss (Inferotemporal). (b) Optical coherence tomography of macula left eye: Faint retinal pigment epithelium elevation consistent with a pigment epithelial detachment. Stable retinal thickening consistent with macular edema (Nasal). Thinning consistent with nerve fiber layer loss (Inferior). Foveal depression present. (c) Large Hollenhorst (cholesterol) plaque seen as a refractile body at a retinal vessel bifurcation along the supratemporal arcade. A couple of other smaller cholesterol plaques are seen surrounding the macular area. Image courtesy Leonid Skorin, Jr., DO, OD, MS, FAAO, FAOCO.

of AMD and glaucoma. A partial retinal artery occlusion was seen on right eye exam with stable Hollenhorst plaques and no new emboli (Figure 10.4c). Several refractile plaques were seen along the inferior temporal artery, with generalized arteriolar narrowing in the right eye. Signs consistent with branch retinal artery occlusion were present on left eye exam. Several refractile plaques were seen in the retina along the superior temporal artery, inferior temporal artery, and nasally in left eye with sclerotic vessels.

The patient was counseled that the visual hallucinations and other color vision disturbances are not real; rather, they are a result of her worsening vision due to ischemia. She was relieved to hear this information; she said she did not believe the hallucinations were real and did not realize that she could be seeing living beings. She is still very concerned about the symptoms increasing, since she had previously been counseled about possible CBS when the purple vision splashes started. She was reassured that if the symptoms worsened and she started seeing new images, another office visit could be necessary to check the integrity of the blood flow to her retina.

Case submitted by Emily Stiles, OMSII, BS. VCOM Carolinas, Spartanburg, SC, USA and James Hall, MD, Retina Consultants of Carolina P.A., Spartanburg, SC, USA.

Case 5

A 92-year-old female presented to the eye clinic for a 6-month intraocular pressure (IOP) check and with complaints of recent-onset visual hallucinations. She claimed she saw a shadowy man standing at her door, despite having lived alone for several years. This figure reminded her of her deceased husband. The figure was stationary and seemed as if he was just watching her. She noted that she did not feel threatened by the figure. She also reported occasions of seeing green and pink flowing colors all throughout her house, but especially in her kitchen. She knew these images were not real and actually enjoyed seeing the colors since she had not seen colors for a long time due to the condition of her eyes. The patient's previous ocular history included end-stage glaucoma, severe dry age-related macular degeneration (AMD), and keratoconjunctivitis sicca (KCS/dry eye) in both eyes. She used latanoprost 0.005% at bedtime and over-the-counter artificial tears as necessary in both eyes. One year ago, her visual acuity was 20/HM (Hand Motion) right eye and 20/CF (Count Fingers) left eye, and 20/CF both eyes. Her visual acuity remained unchanged from her most recent eye examination. She had no reported history of psychiatric illness or of hearing voices. Additionally, the patient was oriented to time, place, and person with appropriate mood and affect. Her IOP was 11 mmHg in each eye. The patient's slit-lamp exam was unchanged, and she was pseudophakic in both eyes. The fundus examination in both eyes showed cup-to-disc ratios of 0.95 with optic nerve atrophy. The optic nerve atrophy was worse in the left eye than the right eye (Figure 10.5). There was geographic atrophy of the macula in the left eye and geographic atrophy to the left of the optic nerve in the right eye (Figure 10.5), both of which are indicative of AMD. This deterioration and

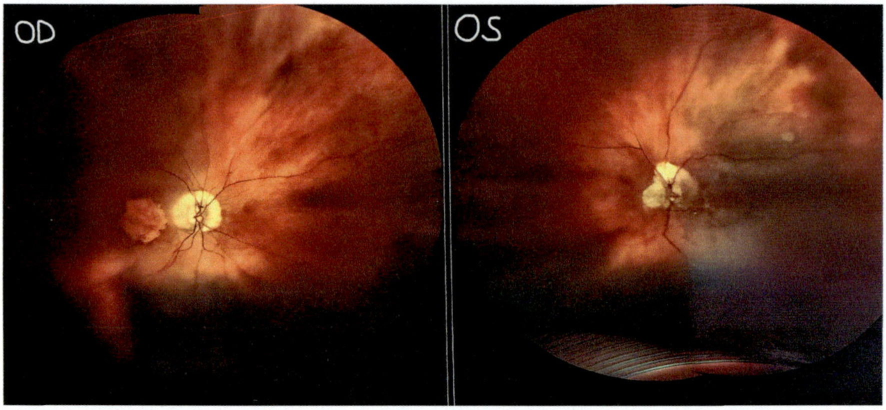

Figure 10.5 Optic nerve atrophy was worse in the left eye (OS) than the right eye (OD). Geographic atrophy of the macula OS and geographic atrophy to the left of the optic nerve in the OD, both of which are indicative of age-related macular degeneration.

long-standing deficiency in both central and peripheral visual acuity are both likely to be the cause of the patient's visual hallucinations. This patient's hallucinations are unique since she exhibited a combination of both static (stationary shadowy man) and dynamic (green and pink colors flowing all throughout her house) imagery.

The patient was reassured that the images resulted from the deterioration in the vision in both her eyes. She was pleased to know that her visual hallucinations had a medical term, Charles Bonnet Syndrome, and that she was not psychologically deteriorating. She did not seem to mind that the hallucinations would probably continue, as her vision loss has progressed significantly and even reiterated her enjoyment of seeing colors again. She was instructed to continue the latanoprost eye drops at bedtime to keep the IOP under control and to continue using the artificial tears as necessary to relieve her symptoms of KCS. She will follow up with her retina specialist for the dry AMD.

Case submitted by Anmol Gosai, OMS-III, MS. Lincoln Memorial University - DeBusk College of Osteopathic Medicine, Harrogate, TN, USA and Jeffrey Holt, MD. Holt Eye Clinic, Hot Springs, AR, USA.

Case 6

An 84-year-old female presented to the eye clinic with complaints of new-onset visual disturbances. She reported seeing various visual hallucinations which she knew were not truly present. The visual hallucinations included snow, rain, food jumping on the plate, water on the floor, people, and pet dogs. The hallucinations were vivid and distressing, as illustrated by an incident where the patient attempted to clean up the perceived water on the floor. Her son noted the unreality of these observations and expressed concern regarding her increasing confusion.

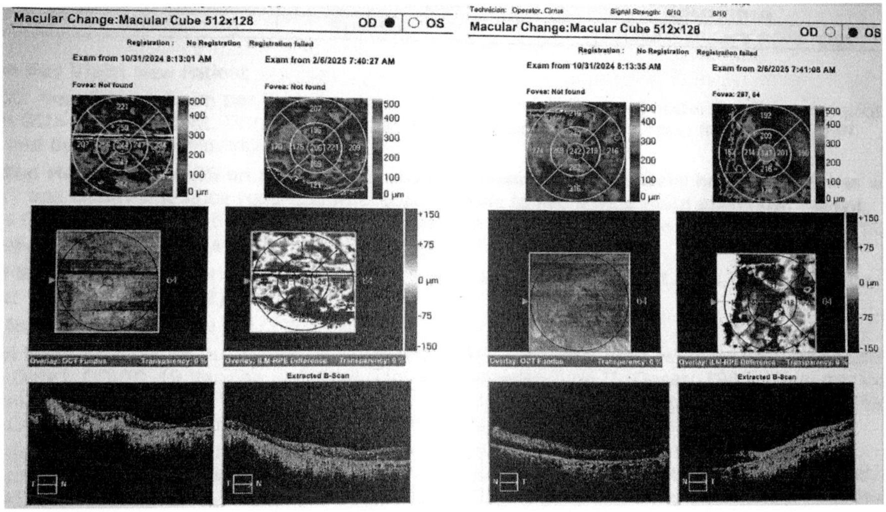

Figure 10.6 Optical coherence tomography of maculas of both eyes—comparison study between October 2024 and February 2025 (right eye (OS)-left images; left eye (OS)-right images). Advanced atrophic macular degeneration both eyes and active choroidal neovascularization left eye.

The patient's pertinent ocular history included neovascular age-related macular degeneration (AMD) with active choroidal neovascularization (CNV) left eye and dry advanced atrophic AMD with subfoveal involvement right eye (Figure 10.6) and bilateral proliferative diabetic retinopathy (PDR). The patient had cataract surgery and pan-retinal photocoagulation (PRP) in both eyes. After receiving PRP treatment, her PDR stabilized. She has been receiving maintenance intravitreal anti-vascular endothelial growth factor injections every eight weeks in the left eye for her AMD and CNV. She is currently not on any ocular medications in either eye. Her visual acuity two months prior was recorded as count fingers at two feet both eyes. However, at her most recent visit her visual acuity had decreased to hand motion both eyes. The patient's family has reported a history of confusion which was also present at the time of her eye clinic visit.

Her intraocular pressure was recorded at 17 mmHg both eyes. The Amsler grid findings showed a central scotoma in the left eye, and the patient was unable to visualize any part of the Amsler grid in the right eye. Her anterior segment exam showed bilateral band keratopathy and a well-centered posterior chamber intraocular lenses. Optic nerve measurement showed a cup-to-disc ratio of 0.2 both eyes with peripapillary atrophy left eye. The right eye fundus exam showed narrowed retinal vessels, retinal pigment epithelial (RPE) atrophy, RPE scarring, and dense PRP in the periphery. The left eye fundus exam showed narrowed retinal vessels with RPE scarring, pigment clumping, and PRP scarring in the periphery.

At the patient's previous eye clinic visit, she described her vision as increasing in darkness and stated, "it's like someone just turned out the lights all of a sudden." Her progressive decline in visual acuity was due to advanced AMD bilaterally and active CNV in the left eye and is the likely contributory factor to the patient's visual hallucinations. The presentation of her visual hallucinations is remarkable in that it displayed both a static and a dynamic component. The patient noticing water on the floor, people, and pet dogs represent the static component while the food jumping on the plate, falling rain, and falling snow, represented the dynamic component.

The diagnosis of Charles Bonnet Syndrome was made based on her clinical presentation and ophthalmic findings. The patient and her family were counseled extensively and reassured that her symptoms were likely due to adaptation to visual deprivation and not indicative of a psychiatric disorder. A four-month follow-up was scheduled to continue managing her AMD and to monitor for any progression of symptoms.

Case submitted by Jasmyne Jenkins, OMS-II, BS. VCOM Carolinas, Spartanburg, SC, USA and John F. Renfro, MD. Retina Consultants of Carolina, P.A., Spartanburg, SC, USA.

Case 7

This client who passed away at 85 years of age was visually impaired as a child with strabismus and had difficulty with focusing that required a strong glasses correction. She would see patterns and would ask others if they had seen that bird, or cat. Her family let this go without further investigation. This expanded to include seeing people in period clothing that she thought of as ghosts. During World War II, she began seeing enemy soldiers in full uniform.

Family members recall her saying that she had keratoconus and was given a choice of having corrective surgery in the 1930s. She decided against surgical treatment as long as she had useful vision. She was diagnosed with glaucoma in her 50s. Her glaucoma progressed to angle-closure glaucoma which resulted in her losing what remained of her usable vision during her 70s and 80s.

Her adult children were at odds regarding the cause of her behavior and images which she claimed she was seeing. One of her medical doctors diagnosed her with dementia based exclusively on the data that she was visualizing these images. During this time, her images became threatening and included such imagery as clowns chasing her and trying to place her into a coffin.

Her daughter believed she was cognitively intact and once asked her what she was seeing. She replied that there were six children sitting around her hassock who seemed to be silently asking for something which she did not know how to provide. The client moved in with her daughter after she began to believe that she had been taken to another house, or one that was a poor duplicate.

She would occasionally try to fight the people she saw invading her daughter's home, which resulted in damage and injury to family members. When she was in her 80s, an ophthalmologist suggested she may have Charles Bonnet Syndrome (CBS), but that there was nothing that could be done about it.

Resources were difficult to find in 2019, but through her daughter's research found and contacted the Charles Bonnet Foundation in Melbourne, Australia, and this author in the U.S.A. who was doing gratis psychology work with individuals with CBS. She received cognitive behavioral therapy which reduced the threatening nature of her visualized images and relieved her depression. Asked how long she had been seeing these images, she replied: "All my life."

Case submitted by: Gary M. Cusick, PhD, Louisville, KY, USA.

Case 8

An 87-year-old Caucasian female presented for a six-month follow-up examination to monitor her neovascular age-related macular degeneration (AMD). She had been living with moderate to advanced AMD for the past five years, which had been slowly progressing over time. During this period, she had been actively receiving anti-VEGF (vascular endothelial growth factor) therapy every six to eight weeks in both eyes to manage the condition. The patient did not have any history of cognitive decline, psychiatric disorders, or other systemic conditions that could lead to visual hallucinations. She was fully oriented to time, place, and person during the examination.

During this eye examination, her visual acuity was found to be worse than from the previous visit. In the right eye (OD), she had vision of counting fingers at 3 feet, compared to 20/400 during the last visit. In her left eye (OS), her vision was 20/200, down from 20/100 previously. Intraocular pressure was measured at OD: 16 mmHg and OS: 17 mmHg using Goldmann applanation tonometry. The patient was pseudophakic in both eyes, and the cup-to-disc ratio was OD: 0.1 and OS: 0.2. Funduscopic examination showed significant macular disruptions in both eyes, consistent with advanced macular degeneration. The fundus showed a large area of dark choroidal hemorrhaging in the central macular region of the right eye (Figures 10.8a, b). The left eye was less drastic with the size of the hemorrhaging but showed evident choroidal changes consistent with neovascular macular degeneration. Optical coherence tomography imaging revealed the presence of choroidal neovascular membranes in both eyes, which had progressed drastically compared to the previous ocular evaluation six months earlier.

At the conclusion of the examination, the patient unexpectedly revealed that she had been experiencing vivid visual hallucinations, which had become increasingly pronounced over the last six months. She described seeing a figure of a younger man, dressed entirely in black clothing, and very tall. She stated he first appeared in her living room. He was standing in the corner of her living room. Despite being able to see his detailed features, such as his face, she found this individual to be a stranger to her. She described the visual hallucination as very realistic and persistent. No matter which room she was in, or what activity she was partaking in this figure of a man was there. In some instances, he would be

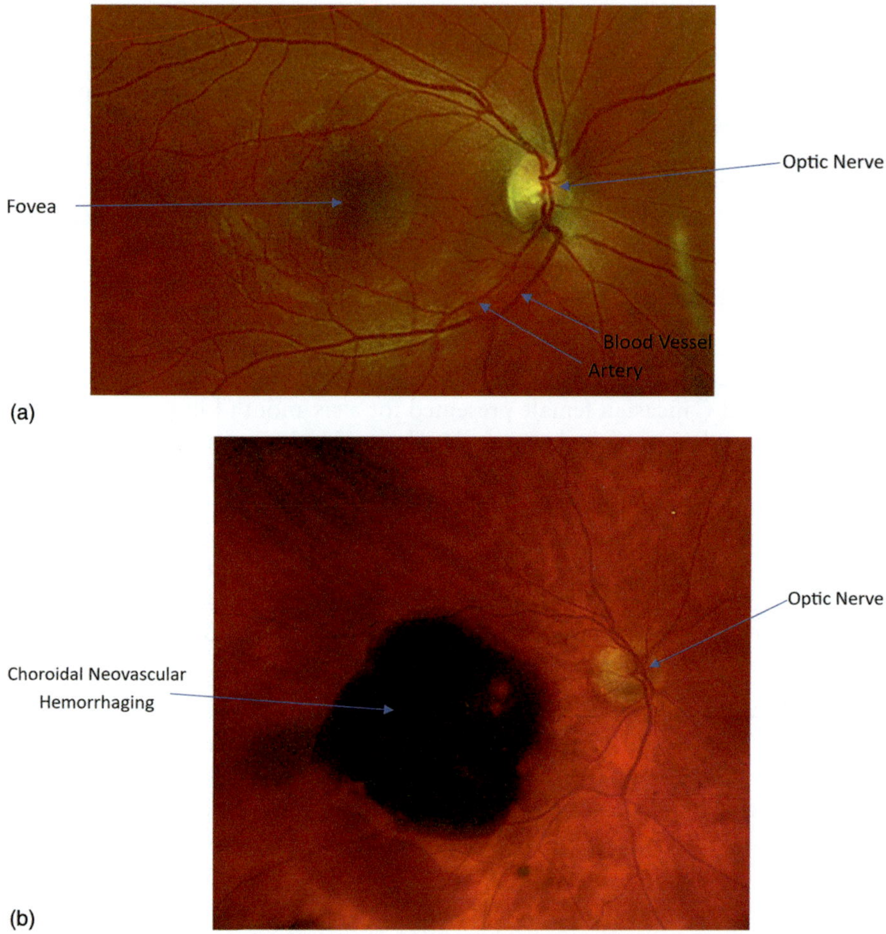

Figure 10.8 (a) Right eye fundus photo of a healthy retina. (b) Right eye choroidal hemorrhage in the macula secondary to uncontrolled neovascular age-related macular degeneration.

pacing back and forth in the room. However, the patient acknowledged that the figure was not physically present, so she was not worried about her personal safety. She expressed concern, nonetheless, fearing that this experience might be a sign of a serious mental illness, given her advanced age.

Upon hearing her concerns, I took the opportunity to educate the patient about the phenomenon of Charles Bonnet Syndrome (CBS). The patient was initially in disbelief, having never heard of such a condition, and was surprised to learn that her experience was not unique. She felt relieved to understand that her visual hallucinations were not indicative of mental decline or an underlying psychiatric disorder. This knowledge helped alleviate her concerns about losing her mental faculties.

To ensure that the patient's healthcare team was well informed about her condition, I took steps to communicate her diagnosis to the appropriate clinicians. A letter was sent to her retinal specialist, detailing the progression of her AMD and the development of the visual hallucinations. The primary care doctor was also informed about CBS and the patient's current experience. As a result, the retinal specialist increased the frequency of her anti-VEGF injections to every four weeks, aiming to manage the progression of the neovascular changes and help improve the patient's overall visual health.

This case highlights the complex relationship between advanced neovascular macular degeneration causing further deterioration of this patient's vision and the occurrence of visual hallucinations. By educating the patient about her condition and ensuring coordination with her healthcare team, a plan was put in place to address both her vision and her mental well-being.

Case submitted by: Andrew Krein, OD, BSc., Devon Eye Clinic, Devon, AB, Canada.

Case 9

A 94-year-old female presented to the eye clinic with complaints of new onset visual disturbances. The patient reported seeing vivid hallucinations, including ghosts, people, floral prints, and colors. She described engaging in conversations with these hallucinated figures and expressed fear that someone might break into her home or harm her. Although she recognized some of the hallucinations as likely unreal, she admitted difficulty distinguishing hallucination from reality. These visual symptoms were further accompanied by headaches.

The patient's ocular history is significant for bilateral dry age-related macular degeneration (AMD) with advanced geographic atrophy, sparing the subfoveal region in both eyes. Her past ocular surgical history includes bilateral cataract extraction. She is currently not on any ocular medications in either eye. On examination, her best corrected visual acuity was counting fingers at 3 feet right eye and 20/250 left eye. The patient was alert and oriented to person, place, and time. She is retired and lives under the care of a caregiver. There is no known psychiatric history, nor any prior history of visual or auditory hallucinations.

Amsler grid testing revealed a central scotoma in both eyes, and the patient noticed distorted lines in the right eye. Intraocular pressures were 11 mmHg right eye, and 12 mmHg left eye. Anterior segment exam was unremarkable except for mild posterior capsular opacification in the left eye and a prior open capsulotomy in the right eye. Optic nerve evaluation revealed an asymmetric cup-to-disc ratio of 0.3 right eye and 0.6 left eye with peripapillary atrophy. Fundus exam of the right eye showed posterior vitreous detachment, extensive geographic atrophy located centrally, temporal drusen, pigment clumping, and retinal pigment epithelial mottling (RPE). Fundus exam of the left eye showed posterior vitreous detachment and temporal RPE mottling.

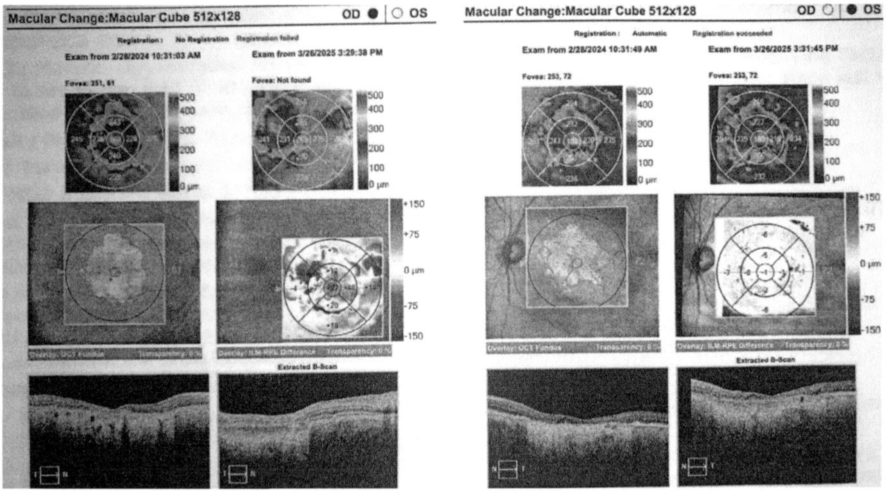

Figure 10.9 Optical coherence tomography of maculas of both eyes—comparison study between February 2024 and March 2025 (right eye (OD)-left images; left eye (OS)-right images). Dry macular degeneration with advanced atrophy, both eyes.

The patient's AMD staging two months prior to her last visit had progressed from intermediate dry AMD to dry AMD with advanced atrophy (Figure 10.9). Her poor visual acuity, particularly in the right eye with the central geographic atrophy, is suspected to have contributed to her visual hallucinations. This patient's hallucinations were remarkable in the sense that it included both a visual and auditory involvement. Although the patient did not perceive the hallucinations as directly addressing her, she still reported having conversations with them. She also exhibited fear and delusional ideation related to the hallucinations

The diagnosis of Charles Bonnet Syndrome was made based on her clinical presentation and ophthalmic findings. The patient was counseled extensively and reassured that her symptoms were likely due to adaptation to visual deprivation and not indicative of a psychiatric disorder. A six month follow-up was scheduled to continue managing her dry macular degeneration and to monitor for any progression of symptoms.

Case submitted by Jasmyne Jenkins, OMS-II, BS. VCOM Carolinas, Spartanburg, SC, USA and John F. Renfro, MD. Retina Consultants of Carolina, P.A., Spartanburg, SC, USA.

Case 10

This case involves an 87-year-old female with macular degeneration who is a resident in an assisted living facility. She is gregarious and lives with a dog that provides her with company and in her mind, safety. She has been open with the other residents of the assisted living facility regarding her visual impairment and

Charles Bonnet Syndrome (CBS). She briefly had other vision impaired residents attend the support group meeting with her. Unfortunately, the staff at the facility do not understand CBS and humor the client as they would a person with dementia.

She will not use a recently bought living room chair because she sees a man she does not know sitting in it throughout the day. Members of the support group and visitors to her room will sit in the chair to demonstrate that there is no danger in doing so. On occasion, she also sees a man and woman on her couch having sex.

For the past seven months an elderly couple who she says claimed to be her parents will enter her room and move her furniture and her extensive collection of bric-a-brac around on a daily basis. She finds this upsetting but admits that later everything has returned to where it was before. Although she does not recognize any of the CBS people/images which she perceives, she says she sees her late second husband at times.

Her son and his wife have attended some support group meetings and have spoken with the group moderator upon occasion. Her son relates that his mother was thought to have agoraphobia prior to moving to the assisted living facility. Older people with visual impairment are more likely to experience anxiety related to falls which may be intensified whenever they walk on uneven surfaces.[2] This may have been a misinterpreted sign due solely to her vision impairment. In my practice of psychology, I have noted that the traditional signs of paranoia and obsessive-compulsive disorder are more evident in visually impaired individuals who are well organized and exercise caution.

Case submitted by: Gary M. Cusick, PhD, Louisville, KY, USA.

Case 11

This case involves a 74-year-old female with retinitis pigmentosa who lives alone with her dog and uses a white cane with a ball end for mobility. She uses a voice-activated assistance device to aid her with time, weather, and other questions that she may have.

Due to multiple emergency hospital visits related to Charles Bonnet Syndrome (CBS), she and her family are well-known to the first responders in her area. She has been prescribed an anticonvulsant, an anxiolytic, and antipsychotic, which makes it difficult for her to wake up. This combination of medications also makes it difficult for her to walk. Furthermore, she complains about problems with short-term memory. Her family life is troubled. She sleeps poorly in a reclining chair. Her blood oxygen level has been recorded as low as 87% (normal range: 92%-100%). A polysomnogram was negative for obstructive sleep apnea.

She experiences CBS images during all waking hours with her eyes open or closed. She understands that the images are not real but refers to "crossing over" when the images appear. Many support group members say: "in the moment" of appearance the image is startlingly real. In addition, she has seen the words "You're Safe" written on a trailer passing by her home where she lives alone. The majority of her images are non-threatening, but occasionally a group of three human images will be "trying to get me." She has a one-eyed Humpty Dumpty whose mouth is stitched up as a repeating image. She may also see naked men in the bathroom.

Her images begin to increase after 2:00 pm, and she needs to take a benzodiazepine when necessary for this. Her anxiety increases when she is alone overnight. A grandson has agreed to stay with her, but he is not always at her home. She can sometimes sleep through the night if her dog remains near her.

Case submitted by: Gary M. Cusick, PhD, Louisville, KY, USA.

Case 12

This 81-year-old lost her sight completely in her right eye due to glaucoma seven years ago, but she retains light perception vision in her left eye. She can be argumentative regarding the reality of the images she perceives and will attempt to talk her caregivers into believing in their existence as she does. She may refuse to answer questions regarding her wellbeing. Her caregiver daughter describes her as "living in a fantasy world."

She has come to believe that she is living in the mountains, which is an immersive or 360° environment. In her case she sees the mountains when she thinks she is looking out the window. She also sees a floating map, which would fall into the pattern type of her Charles Bonnet Syndrome (CBS). She is frequently observed isolating and talking to herself. She tries to entertain the human images she sees. This interaction gives her the feeling of being able to see again. She sometimes believes that the human images she visualizes intend to harm her. She is overwhelmed by noise. She has been prescribed antidepressants, antipsychotics and anxiolytics, which must be administered by her caregiver in her food as suggested by her medical doctor.

Her CBS has had a negative impact on her family. Her husband believes she has lost her mind. Her daughter has accepted the role of her primary caregiver. Unfortunately, her daughter is now showing signs of caregiver stress. Her daughter feels exhausted, feels stuck, sleeps poorly, is gaining weight, and cries intermittently. To date her daughter has received no counseling and her preexisting medical conditions have gotten worse.

The health and safety of the caregiver is as essential as for the health and safety of the person with CBS. Caregiver Syndrome is a real concern in many of these situations. Most research on this subject addresses the caregivers who are responsible for individuals with heart disease, cancer, and other non-vision related issues. The American Medical Association offers a caregiver assessment online for those in need.[3]

Case submitted by: Gary M. Cusick, PhD, Louisville, KY, USA.

REFERENCES

1. Cushing H, *The Life of Sir William Osler*, Vol II. London: Oxford University Press; 1940:295.
2. Hashemi A, et al., *Sci Report.* 2024. doi:10.1038/s41598-024-52389-6
3. Home | HealthInAging.org [Internet]. Healthinaging.org. 2019. https://www.healthinaging.org/. Accessed 8/9/2025.

Index

Pages in *italics* refer to figures.

For Product Safety Concerns and Information please contact our
EU representative GPSR@taylorandfrancis.com Taylor & Francis
Verlag GmbH, Kaufingerstraße 24, 80331 München, Germany